ADDICTION EXPLORATION 2-IN-1 COMBO

THE WEIGHT OF ADDICTION + SUBSTANCE ABUSE,
OPIOIDS-UNDERSTANDING ADDICTION & HOW
TO FIGHT BACK

MILTON HARRISON

© Copyright 2020 - All rights reserved.

It is not legal to reproduce, duplicate, or transmit any part of this document in either electronic means or in printed format. Recording of this publication is strictly prohibited and any storage of this document is not allowed unless with written permission from the publisher except for the use of brief quotations in a book review.

CONTENTS

THE WEIGHT OF ADDICTION

Introduction	7
1. What Is Addiction?	11
2. How Addiction Happens	31
3. Understanding the Past in Order to Build a Future	44
4. A Balanced and Purposeful Life is a Sober Life	53
5. Developing New Habits	70
6. Staying Active to Move Forward	84
7. In Review	93
8. Conclusion	104
References	107

SUBSTANCE ABUSE, OPIOIDS

Introduction	113
1. The Unavoidable Human Experience	117
2. Addiction and Stigma	130
3. Opioids and Why be Skeptical	140
4. Signs of Addiction and How to Notice them Early	161
5. If You Need Them, Use Them Responsibly	178
6. Medication as Treatment	189
7. Seek the Help of Others	200
8. TMC and Other Natural Treatments	214
Afterword	227
References	235

THE WEIGHT OF ADDICTION

ACTIVITIES, HABITS, AND TREATMENTS TO PRODUCE CHANGE

INTRODUCTION

"It does not matter how slowly you go as long as you do not stop."

— CONFUCIUS

Freedom is the greatest motivator. People have started revolutions, wars, and movements because of this universal truth. Humanity has scaled higher levels of education and knowledge in order to achieve it, for true liberation that can only be obtained through insight. Freedom has a variety of meanings to different people. This personal, individual definition depends on one's background, and the reasoning behind their desire for it.

Addiction, in itself, is a restriction of that freedom. It weighs you down and creates a vast array of difficulties preventing you from becoming the best you can be. Perhaps, in your situation, you want to be a better student and take your grades and academic priorities seriously, but you just can't seem to get it down. This is not because you have any literacy issues, and it certainly is not because you are lacking in intelligence. When you took the time to figure out why, it turned out you had an addiction to playing video games. While this may seem trivial, it is far from that; in fact, there is great importance there. You find, after doing some self-discovery, that you can hardly function without playing video games. It has begun to take a toll on other parts of your life: socializing, family, and interests in general. It is scary to admit, but the facts remain.

Maybe your personal experience is that you can't go a day without smoking. There has been justification in the past because you don't smoke a pack a day, but you just are not able to stop. Whenever you need to cope with something, you reach for a cigarette. When stress is introduced to your life, you go for a cigarette again. Recognizing this pattern is incredibly important, but it still is only a first step.

Whether your addiction is drugs, alcohol, gambling, watching pornography, exercising, or even eating, you must come to the realization that it hinders you from maximizing your potential. Addiction weighs you down.

The possibilities of a life free from the downward spirals and destruction of addiction are endless. This book and the lessons within will expose you to the benefits of living a life without the restrictions and pain that can come from the cycles of an addict. and can serve as a guide for your entire journey. A life after addiction will bring you the opportunity to have better relationships, healthy and productive hobbies, and self-fulfillment. Every step you take on your journey to a new, fresh, revitalized life is worth it. *You* are worth it.

During the course of this journey, you will learn how to alter your perspectives to regain a healthy outlook on life, and the correct images of both yourself and the life you are leading. You will be uplifted and challenged, but never judged. You have either been a victim of extreme judgement, or you have known someone who has experienced that; both are far too prevalent in the lives of those going through the recovery process. Above all, you are a good person who has realized the direction their life was headed, and mustered the strength to make a change. With that change, that life altering choice, you began a series of forward-moving steps that will gradually lead you into a life that is bright and filled with potential.

This book is for everyone who can relate to the challenging situations we just laid out. This book is for all of us who struggled, or still struggle with drugs, alcohol, gambling, shopping, eating, exercising, or whatever addiction has eaten away at both your joy and life. I can promise you that this book will provide you with the knowledge, tools, and techniques you need to overcome addiction. This set of guidelines will change the way you look at life. You will know what it is like to be empowered with the courage to take control back by casting off the shackles of addiction. If you are struggling with addiction in any way, this book provides you with a step-by-step guide on how to break free from it. You will learn activities that you can get involved in to free yourself, as well as habits that you have to break or relearn.

The information that will be covered is an in-depth guide on this type of dependence and the ways in which you can overcome it to move forward into a life of purpose. This information is not a substitute for medical attention, and neither is it a replacement for the recommended therapy or support groups deemed necessary for one's journey to a life free of addiction. If you are worried or anxious about the changes you will have to make in your life, remember that you don't have to do it all at once. You can take it slowly. In fact, it is both suggested and healthy to have a steady, healthy approach. You do not want to rush into these kinds of changes because it will most likely drain you of whatever drive you have. As long as you are consistent and committed, you will achieve your goal. You will break free of your addiction to discover a full life on the other side.

If you want to free yourself from the weight of addiction, you need to properly understand what that truly means, what the definition is in all its forms. The first step to free yourself from a life beholden to that addictive act or substance is to understand what the cause or the root is. Beginning with the first chapter, and for the remainder of our time together, you will start to unravel the pain, challenges, and depth that exist within the life you are trying to leave behind. With trust, inspired action, and your capable strength there is nothing you cannot achieve, including a life of sobriety.

1

WHAT IS ADDICTION?

A few years ago, I heard about a boy, a young man now, who lost both his parents in an unfortunate accident. He was in college when it happened. When he heard about it, this young man turned to alcohol to cope with his grief. The more time passed, the more he would use drinking to mask even more pain. He eventually developed such a strong dependency on it that he started skipping classes, stopped turning in homework, and lost the friends he had through continued isolation and drastic personality changes. As the difficulties and consequences piled up, he reached a point where he had to drop out of college. It wasn't an overnight change, but his life was overtaken at a gradual, wretched pace.

It has become far too commonplace for people to hear stories like this cautionary tale of people whose lives have taken a turn for the worse - or ended - because of addiction. Maybe you are even one of the afflicted whose lives have changed to these extreme degrees. Perhaps a similar experience followed that same steady destruction to where you have lost your job. The damages are far-reaching, spreading to relationships, your sense of autonomy, your finances but you can gain it all back. It takes work and dedication, but it can happen. *You* can make it happen but not without taking action.

Through the ages, humanity has struggled with addictions to various substances such as alcohol, cannabis, and cocaine, to name some of the better known offenders. The dissuasion from intoxication common is an occurrence across all societies in different eras. In fact, some cultures restricted the use of some substances to specific rituals or events. For the ancient Aztecs, alcohol served a ceremonial purpose and its consumption outside of such purpose was punishable by death. Even ancient philosophers and physicians recognized the possibility of addiction, as well as the dangers of substances such as alcohol or opium. Aristotle recognized the harmful effects of alcohol consumption on pregnant women and studied the side effects of alcohol withdrawal.

Addiction became an even more prominent issue upon industrialization, colonization, and globalization. As international trade became more possible, alcohol and other substances were made available for the population. In the 18th Century, Benjamin Rush, an American physicist, posited that the lack of self-control by drinkers was caused by the drink rather than the drinkers. In the 19th Century, medical journals were created for the purpose of studying addiction. This study was influenced by the opiate addiction that ravaged America and Europe. No matter the time period, the same story was being told with different characters. Each passing century saw the world grow a little smaller, a little closer together, until cultural exports were reaching places never before thought possible. While this introduced many positive aspects into the international scene, when a substance arrived that held the addictive potential as the previously mentioned examples, the results were usually a documented pattern.

In recent years, addiction has continued to move towards the forefront of both policy and public opinion, with a focus on substance abuse being the primary link to addiction. According to the World

Drug Report released by the United Nations Office on Drugs and Crime (UNODC) in 2019, about 35 million people worldwide suffer from a form substance use disorder. The report estimates the number of opioid users worldwide to be 53 million, putting the figures higher than that of the other types of drug use disorder. These figures resonate with even more impact when you consider the number of Americans that suffer from substance use disorder. The National Survey on Drug Use and Health (NSDUH) reported that 19.7 million Americans struggled with substance use disorder in 2017. Considering the exponential growth of the afflicted, every day the issue becomes more dire.

Addiction can be defined by some as the abnormal dependence of a person on an activity or a habit-forming substance to the point where abstinence from the cause of the addiction inflicts negative symptoms. Addiction is a rather complex condition. Despite its harmful and disproportionately negative consequences on the mind and body of an individual suffering from addiction, it maintains its hold on such a person. When the brain is constantly exposed to addictive stimuli such as gambling, the use of drugs, the rush or high that comes with playing video games, and a variety of other possible circumstances, it begins to crave the rewards that are associated with such activities. Addiction to substances progress from use to abuse to dependence: this is how the body comes to require the substance to function.

There isn't a switch that suddenly flips, turning someone from a non-user into a user. The process usually goes unrecognized for some time, especially when the overuse is an effective masking agent for whatever the person is trying to escape. That bond between not feeling pain - physical or emotional - begins to create that belief within the mind that without the substance or act, the pain will come flooding back. Addressing the subject of addiction is never a simple thing; in fact, when done correctly, it painstakingly reveals layers upon layers of introspection before real healing can begin. Without recognizing the many areas that impact the intensity of the addiction, you are not going to be following the best path to freedom, peace, and true remedy.

Addiction may sometimes be mistaken for misuse, especially on the topic of substance consumption. The two concepts are different, despite sharing some similarities. A person may misuse drugs by taking more than was prescribed by a qualified doctor or physician but they may not, in fact, be addicted to the drugs. In such a scenario, addiction happens when the individual cannot do without the consumption of the drugs, in an even higher quantity. Oftentimes, misuse of substances leads to addiction. The crossing of that line usually occurs when the misuse ends up "treating" another symptom: pain medication to mentally avoid dealing with financial burdens; steroids meant for inflammation used to try a back-alley way of bulking up. While the initial medication, or substance, was obtained for a health-conscious, medically-approved reason with specific instructions, the methods in which it was used created the right environment for addiction to thrive.

A person suffering from addiction may not realize what they are going through. Addiction to certain activities or substances can blur a person's sense of self-reflection. It is therefore important for one to know the common symptoms of a person struggling with addiction of any kind. By taking the time to identify both the stages of addiction as well as the underlying factors behind those stages, you are allowing yourself the chance to heal - maybe for the first time in your life.

When dealing with the surrounding circumstances as well as the addiction itself, it is incredibly important to remember that there is no singular answer or approach. You will see this repeated often throughout these pages, and for good reason. We are all vastly diverse individuals - whether we are talking about siblings, spouses, or strangers. It is precisely because of these differences that there cannot be an unchanging, concrete way to handle the road to recovery for someone struggling with the challenges of addiction. While there will be many different lessons and points made as we continue, every single word is meant to be adapted to your personal situation.

Perhaps there is a section that speaks particularly to you; do not be afraid to spend extra time on those areas. Take extensive notes. Use this book as source material for further research. However you go about it, you should always give yourself the freedom to experience this guideline in a way that you can relate to. In the same way, there might be parts that you do not feel any connection with, nor do you feel it is advantageous to your recovery program. That is also perfectly okay! You are building a new life, so you and your support group will know the best methods and areas which need the most focus.

Personalize everything as you can! *You* are the focus. *You* have the liberty to adjust and adapt where needed, as long as your health and well-being are the priority.

SYMPTOMS OF ADDICTION

There are many indicators that a person is suffering from addiction. It is important to recognize the signs of possible dependence in order to properly work on yourself. A person suffering from some form of substance disorder may develop a sudden lack of self-control, or they may find that they are unable to stop the addictive behavior; these are examples of symptoms. With every decision you make along this journey, you are being given another tool that will be vital in having a full, well-rounded life.

The subsequent paragraphs will discuss some possible symptoms of addiction.

Lack of Control

A major symptom of addiction is a lack of self-control. You may find that you want to reduce your consumption of alcohol, or maybe you want to limit the hours you spend playing video games, but you can't.

Even though you regret it, you just cannot stop yourself from engaging in that activity or consuming that substance. Feeling like you have lost control is a major cause of addiction, as well as the groundwork for other signs of addiction. Awareness of self and being able to cultivate self-control is an essential part of freedom.

It is important to uncover the difference between *willpower* and *self-control*. A commonly accepted concept within the realm of psychology is that willpower leads to - or is a catalyst to - self-control. In 2011, Americans considered the chief reason they didn't achieve their goals to be directly attributed to their willpower[1]. In that same vein of thinking, losing self-control will gradually erode the strength of that will. By viewing it from the perspective of the two being in a balanced, symbiotic relationship, you can be aware enough to sense when something is off with either - or both.

Loss of Interest in Other Activities

Oftentimes, people who struggle with addiction find it difficult to maintain or build up interests. This is usually because, over time, the only activities they would engage in would involve the harmful substance or activities that fuel their addiction. They tend to neglect such activities because they neither encourage the activity nor the use of the substance. If you constantly put off recreational, educational, or social activities because you want to use a substance or engage in an activity that you are dependent on, you are most likely addicted. This loss of interest in non-addiction related activities sometimes destroys the relationships in your life.

In actuality, what occurs is not so much a *loss* of interest, but more a transfer. That time in your life prior to when addiction was in charge, you found joy and that interest in the activity itself, including the actions, the social aspect, or simply being able to relax and separate from stress. Once that dependence crept in, you found those same areas of fulfillment, but *solely* in the addiction. You simply moved where your enthusiasm was, and a part of recovery and learning how to live a new life means finding a way to move it back.

This is also a pertinent subject to bring up concerning the recovery process itself. A loss of interest is a very common red flag as an indication of a deeper issue, but the subject of "interests" will also come into play later. Consider now, as a starter, what activities or hobbies have drawn your interest as you began your recovery, and now wherever you are in your timeline? Life is about more than survival, as you are discovering, and part of that journey is enjoyment.

Negative Effects on Social Life and Relationships

Addiction has negative consequences on your life, this has been a frequently discussed concept already. People who struggle with this disorder may lash out at others, especially at those in their lives who have noticed their dependency on substances and/or activities that are negatively impacting their lives. They may also experience mood swings and massive blows to their self-esteem. This is because they often feel guilt about their addiction but are unable to stop themselves. If you are going through this, you are not alone.

It is the secrecy that tends to increase the negative effects on you and those around you. There is a significant burden that rests on the mind when you have to literally split your life in two: one portion that must effectively hide the usage while still maintaining it, and the other part that has to act normal in social situations. Trying to juggle these partitions of self becomes exhausting, and can also create a sense of paranoia. If *you* know everything that is going on, then every action or word someone says to you could be misconstrued as suspicion or accusation. This puts the addicted person on a constant defensive stance, leading to more exhaustion, and eventually to the lashing out we discussed above.

Significant Energy Spent on Secrecy

Addiction is a truly tiring condition that leaves a person feeling drained. You are constantly hiding your addiction from people because you do not want them to know what you are going through. You may even become paranoid when they start asking questions about your loss of weight, or any other obvious physical signs of your addiction, mostly because it is connected to your use. Addiction and secrecy are dangerous because the continued consumption of the addictive substance or engagement in the habit-forming behavior often has negative consequences. Secrecy while attempting to stop using drugs or alcohol can lead to death.

Increased Tendency to Take Risks

When a person is addicted, they will do almost anything to get their "fix." The possibility of taking risks increases on two fronts: the need to access the activity or substance, and the need to use or engage without being caught. People struggling with addiction push their limits every time they use the substance or engage in the activity they are addicted to. Have you ever come up with an elaborate scheme to avoid getting caught while using?

The next stage of this is what ends up creating the longevity of an addiction, and that is scheming to get away with it. When you manage to avoid consequence the first time you take a risk - stealing, lying, etc. - the reward can be as immediate and fulfilling as the substance itself. You are aware that in order to continue this system of using, the act you just undertook will most likely have to be repeated. Because this is an established fact, realizing that you got away with it will create a false sense of being untouchable, thus that may be the trigger for the increase in risk. Remember that addiction will *never* plateau, which is why it is not a viable treatment and is simply a mask. Every rung you climb on the risk ladder will lead upwards to another more difficult, more damaging one, until you either fall or begin to climb back down.

Withdrawal Symptoms

The most difficult part of addiction is quitting. The thing about addiction is that cessation of the use of the substance or cessation of the activity itself causes emotional and physical trauma. You may have tried to quit feeding your addiction once or twice but you could not get through nausea, anxiety, sweats, and other withdrawal symptoms. It is not easy to overcome addiction by oneself, especially substance addiction.

Just like the patterns that assisted in getting you to this point, once you start to give in it will naturally become easier. This can also create a cycle, one that emerges each time you consider getting clean. It is okay to admit fear when you consider the true depth of withdrawals, but it is also necessary to know the good health and positive promises that come from getting through it. There has to be belief, both in yourself and in the process, for it to be effective and for you to be willing to undertake the challenge.

Tolerance

The more a person consumes substances, or engages in behaviors that are addictive, the greater the amount they need to appease the body's learned appetite. For example, when a person keeps overeating, their brain releases dopamine to reinforce the connection between food and pleasure, thus causing them to eat even more, even more often. When they continue that cycle, their brain continues releasing high amounts of dopamine. The body recognizes an improper balance going on, and tries to repair the irregularity by regulating the amount of dopamine and starts producing less. This becomes an issue because their brain still requires a certain amount of dopamine to function properly. The body makes up for the lesser than normal dopamine by causing them to crave food, knowing from experience that this increased intake can rectify the situation.

In effect, you are putting your mind and body at war with one another, and sometimes within the same factions. Both systems are dedicated to balance, but as these distortions of the status quo continue, they will be forced to adjust. The body is a truly incredible machine, and when a foreign operation is introduced the internal procedures are thrown off kilter.

TYPES OF ADDICTION

Although most people consider substance addiction to refer to a singular idea or singular kind of addiction, there are two recognized types of addiction: Behavioral Addiction and Substance Addiction. Both of these two versions affect individuals differently, as with the other symptoms of the affliction itself. One person may have a tendency to turn to one substance and one substance only, while another ends up developing an addiction to both a behavior and a substance, while a third example could show a person having a completely different experience altogether with addiction. When dealing with something as deeply complex as the subject of addiction, it is important to recognize the fluidity of the impacts. There is a required respect that comes with the territory, and in this instance you must respect the impossibility in having a singular approach to this issue.

Because of this, let's observe the different variations that occur when discussing addiction:

Behavioral Addiction

Behavioral Science experts determined that anything that is capable of causing dependence through stimulation can be an addiction. When behaviors become compulsory and obligatory, they inch toward being under the umbrella definition of an addiction. Behavioral dependency may be harder to notice than substance addiction because it is incredibly common to mistake this variation for an obsessive interest. While you could be considered a "super fan" or over-the-top, when the actions fall under a more social category, they can be seen as simply habits that many people engage in. Most people would not bat an eyelid at someone who is always on the internet, or someone who is always shopping. When someone's hygiene and self-image begin to suffer from a dependence on the internet, or when severe financial disruption occurs due to one's obsession with shopping, those are red flags.

Behavioral addictions such as internet browsing, overeating, shopping, gambling, sex and pornography, overworking, and many more, are too often seen as outside the realm of addiction because the individual is addicted to the particular behavior or the feeling attached to it. Unfortunately, in these cases, the problem isn't seen until it reaches an extreme level. Just like any other disease, addiction can be fatal or have permanent damage if left until the advanced stages.

The National Council on Problem Gambling reported that more than 2 percent of Americans are addicted to gambling. The 5th edition of the Diagnostic and Statistical Manual of Mental Disorders (DSM-V) recognizes gambling addiction as the only non-substance addiction. There are still disagreements as to whether behaviors and habits can be causes of addiction. This is because there are still debates about which activities can become addictive, and there is yet to be an agreed-upon point at which behaviors become addictions. Although, as stated above, the stance commonly taken by professionals is that if a behavior *can* be classified as causing dependence, it can also be seen as an addictive action.

The lack of peer-reviewed scientific evidence is the reason for its exclusion from the DSM-V. Regardless of the lack of scientific diagnosis, many people struggle with behavioral addictions. People struggling with behavioral addiction often find that their relationships with people are negatively affected. More often than not, they may have serious financial repercussions and problems.

While it is known that there is a vilified stigma around the term *addiction*, it is important to also recognize when real, presenting issues of dependence arise in the behavioral form that they are often shrugged off. There seems to be a subconscious need to rate the types of addiction, and therefore rank where you prioritize them. Drugs and other substances are more mainstream in their coverage, so when they are present in the real world the reaction is more sympathetic. On the other hand, when the presentation is on the side of behavior, the reaction is much less understanding. In fact, I have heard reasonings to dismiss these cases due to the fact that they would distract from "actual addiction problems."

Dealing with addiction demands compassion, and part of that is the removal of these dangerous and destructive stereotypes and assumptions. There is a good chance that an addict has not felt much acceptance during their struggles, and by viewing their real pain and challenges in an unsympathetic manner will do untold damage to an already lost person.

Substance Addiction

This is the commonly accepted type of addiction. Substance addiction is the dependence on any chemical intoxicant or substance. Addiction to substances such as alcohol, cocaine, cannabis, and opioids have a very high chance of causing dependency. The Diagnostic and Statistical Manual of Mental Disorders (DSM-V) recommends the term substance use disorder when dealing with substance addiction.

The DSM-V classifies drugs into ten separate classes and recognizes substance use disorders that could arise from the use of these drugs. The ten classes of drugs are thus: alcohol; tobacco; cannabis; inhalants; opioids; hallucinogens (such as LSD, phencyclidine, and others); stimulants (such as cocaine, and amphetamine-type substances); hypnotics, sedatives, and anxiolytics; caffeine; and unknown substances. It is important to not simply pass over that information because, as we discussed earlier, the subject of addiction - any type of addiction - requires both seeing the depth of information at hand and the importance of understanding the different variations rather than generalizing.

Substance addiction often has physical and psychological impacts upon the individual. In regards to the physical consequences, constant consumption of alcohol could cause inflammation of the liver, damage to the pancreas, permanent brain dysfunction, and lengthy list of other physical harms. Addiction to alcohol could also put a person at a higher risk of pneumonia, along with the damaging of the heart and liver. Pregnant women who remain addicted to alcohol put their unborn child at risk of having Fetal Alcohol Syndrome. Fetal alcohol syndrome (FAS) is a condition that occurs in children who were exposed to alcohol while in the womb. It causes growth problems and brain damage.

In 2017, over 180,000 people died from alcohol disorder, making it the highest cause of death among other substance use disorders. Despite this fact, and that the statistics have been available for some time, it remains incredibly difficult to maintain distance from alcohol in today's world. Not only that, but the reaction in social situations to someone who no longer partakes is rarely positive, and usually uncomfortable. The widespread availability of alcohol creates a dangerous environment to the members of society who suffer from the affliction.

The psychological consequences of substance addiction revolve around mental health. Many people who are addicted to substances are diagnosed with mental disorders. Substance addiction causes changes in the brain, and these changes could lead to depression, hallucinations, anxiety, and other problems. In the same line of thought, when dealing with those who have a long-term addiction, the withdrawals alone could lead to these disorders. While the full impact of this type of continued abuse remains unknown, what we do know shows a need for as much healing as possible, while realizing the serious nature of the circumstance.

Similarities Between the Types of Addiction

Generally, behavioral and substance addiction share similar reactions from the brain. In both types of addiction, continued use or engagement causes the brain to require more in order to avoid withdrawal symptoms. Tolerance is a shared result of both types of addiction. Another similarity is the general lack of interest in activities other than those which encourage their addiction. For example, someone who is addicted to cocaine will most likely lose interest in anything that is not cocaine. The same goes for someone who is addicted to watching television; they will most likely be hooked to their TVs, rather than anything else.

People who are addicted to substances or activities tend to lose self-control. This lack of self-control is a major driving force for the two types of addiction. This loss of self-control is evident in the need to continue using, despite the negative consequences of addiction in a person's life.

Differences Between the Types of Addiction

The major difference between substance addiction and behavioral addiction is that, in the former, the individual is addicted to a substance while the latter sees the individual addicted to a particular behavior or the feeling that comes with indulging in such behavior.

The physical signs of substance addiction are often absent in cases of behavioral addiction. For instance, some physical signs that indicate the use of cannabis and other cannabis-containing substances are red eyes and dry mouth. These physical signs would not be present in a person struggling with exercise addiction.

Another variation is the approach that is usually taken in regards to these two, as we briefly touched on earlier. Since substance addiction is the more visible or recognizable of the two, it is given more validity compared to a behavioral type of addiction. While it is important to understand the issue of addiction as a whole, it cannot be done without also seeing the individual impacts and characteristics associated with each specific case. Above all, never get to a point where you only see an issue or a disease, especially with yourself! The people behind those labels and variations are the focus, *you* are the focus. Well being, health, and stability, those are the goals, no matter what kind of an addiction you are dealing with.

THE BIOLOGY OF ADDICTION: HOW DOES IT WORK?

If you are struggling with addiction, you may have tried to quit, and if it did not take then it would have been difficult for you. You may have lost your friends or family, maybe even your job or a scholarship. You are not happy about the way you are but you don't know how to stop. Why is it so difficult to quit? Why do you keep going back, even though you know better?

We've discussed some of the mental aspects of addiction, but when it comes to biology, it is a compilation of a few different systems. Your mind understands at least some of the danger you continue to put yourself in, but that occurs while your body is demanding that you satiate the craving. When that isn't fulfilled, you experience both physical and emotional trauma from the sudden deficiency of the substance in your body. When this cycle is repeated enough, using the addiction as treatment, the mind begins to alter its stance and the voices of reason become dimmer. After a while you will have your body and mind working together in a continuous structure designed around addiction fulfillment.

The use of medicine for the treatment of addiction seems counterintuitive to some but scientists have shown that treatments can control the need for substances. Having a dependency is a long-lasting condition affecting both mind and body, and that is why people who successfully quit are never fully free from the danger of returning to addiction. The biology of this process proves that people need more than just willpower and determination to overcome these challenges and afflictions. The more addicted or dependent a person is to a substance or an activity, the more changes happen within the brain. It takes a lot of work and time for the brain to return to its normal state and, unfortunately, in some cases there really is no going back.

Your body is incredibly adept at healing: from bones to muscle and even types of nerves will regrow, sometimes stronger than before. The brain, however, is a much more fragile system. The toll your body undergoes during the addiction usually reveals itself in time, and when you begin to repair yourself, the healing will show in your appearance as well. Your mind is much harder to fix, if it can be fixed at all. This is why there is a sense of urgency when it comes to entering recovery, because each day spent in the cycle of damage could be the day something unfixable ends up being harmed.

The power of addiction is in its ability to control and oftentimes destroy the key areas of the brain involved with our survival. The constant use of drugs can damage the prefrontal cortex, the part of the brain that controls decision-making. As a result of this, people are unable to make the decision to stop using drugs even though they know they consume too much, even though their act of using is damaging their relationships with people, and despite the fact that they realize that they will eventually have to steal to buy drugs, if that isn't already the case.

This damage to the regions of your brain can also cause you to live in multiple worlds. What this means is that you have to justify your actions to yourself somehow, and the further into the addiction you go, the more you need to condone. Because you cannot fully admit the extent of your situation - because then you would have to address it - you need to go to more and more extremes to warrant the actions you take. From this comes an imaginary world of "one day" where all your good choices reside.

One day you'll come clean to everyone, but not now.

One day you will find a way to work through all these issues, but today you just can't.

A healthy brain rewards healthy activities and behaviors such as moderate exercising, swimming, reading, or bonding with people. When a person engages in such productive and robust activities, the brain motivates them to repeat the activities; the brain is incentivizing, really. A healthy mind functions properly, even in times of emergency or danger. Having this positive, strong, active perspective on life prompts immediate reaction to dangerous situations in order to protect you.

In situations that may have negative consequences, the prefrontal cortex decides on the course of action. But when the brain is affected by addiction, especially to an addictive substance, its normal processes can be affected. Addiction can make the danger-sensing parts of the brain go haywire; thus, causing anxiety, stress, and nervousness even when the individual is not using. Addiction can also control the part of the brain responsible for rewarding behaviors, and cause an individual to want more. When people are addicted to substances or behaviors, they often turn to using them to stop from feeling bad, rather than for pleasure.

In fact, over time, the user can experience a "new normal" where life has switched, in a sense. They have used so much that their time spent under the influence now feels normal, while the time in sobriety is uncomfortable and surreal, considering it is usually spent on the search for another fix. While this is not always the case, getting to this point can have lasting effects on how someone views the world.

Scientists have been unable to pinpoint exactly why some people get addicted while others do not. According to the National Institutes of Health, the risk of addiction has a tendency to increase in people whose parents are alcoholics or drug addicts. Addiction is sometimes caused by multiple genes. While scientists have been unable to determine the precise genetic cause, research has shown that genes may have an influence regarding substance use. In fact, scientists have estimated the influence of genetics in causing addiction occurs in nearly 60 percent of studied cases. It is important to note that the risk of addiction from certain genes does not mean that every member of a family will be affected. This is a fluctuating science that has very little concrete information at this time, and as such should be handled with both care and patience.

Our genes, however, are not the only factor that increases the risk of possible addiction. People who grew up around addicts are also at a higher chance of becoming addicts themselves. Also, children who come from homes that normalize physical and mental abuse are at higher risk of becoming addicted to substances. The earlier a person starts consuming substances such as alcohol and cocaine, the greater the likelihood of addiction.

In essence, when someone spends their formative years in an environment of fear or trauma, the desire to escape this reality will be present from an early stage. While the reasons for the turn to addiction differs from person to person, the core desire is to remove oneself from the issues around them, to escape. Consistent immersion in such a negative space from a young age can certainly bring about these circumstances of addiction more expediently, and at a more intense level.

THE EVOLUTION OF ADDICTION

Addiction can be viewed from an evolutionary perspective, as well, in order to discover the causes of substance abuse. This approach to dependency also supports psychological treatment alongside medication, as it aims to prevent substance use disorders. There is significant research that points to the co-evolution of mammalian brains and psychotropic plants, plants that affect a person's mind. Thus, human brains and these specific types of plants affected one another during the process of evolving; these plants were not as potent as they are now, and the human brain developed receptors for the plants.

Evidence for this coevolution is the body's development of defenses against over-toxicity, such as vomiting reflexes.

The early form of humans would collect plants and, as time passed, they learned that some of these plants caused euphoric reactions or contained healing properties. For the plants that had a more intoxicating effect, people would harvest those more than others. Extensive research has shown that in order to cope on an evolutionary scale, there developed an arms race, of sorts. The plant would evolve stronger chemical compounds to dissuade humans from consuming them, and the people would develop a tolerance or learn how to regulate the impact[2]. Some possible examples of this, according to several botanical experts, are nicotine, morphine, and atropine, to name just a few[3].

The human brain is vulnerable to addiction because the parts of the brain that regulate behavior are based on chemical transmitters. It is therefore unsurprising that people get addicted to substances which can easily stimulate the system. The susceptibility of the human brain to addiction is proof that you are not weak because of your addiction, and there are other factors that increase the risk of addiction. When people begin to look at the entire study of dependency from an evolutionary standpoint, they are closer to understanding how to remedy and prevent addiction without only treating the symptoms.

Whether it is evolutionary, genetic, or from a different origin altogether, it is important to think of addiction from every possible perspective. The more you understand the underlying causations, the damage done and subsequent healing, the more this information enables you to be constructive. Recovery is a process, whether it is for you or a loved one. There is a person behind the judgement and vilified stigmas, a person who has seen the lowest places that humanity can go, a person who both deserves and needs love as well as the respect needed to take the time to understand their perspective.

Addiction is a brain condition which has a greater effect worldwide on more people than we are willing to admit. It comes in many forms and, until people address it, it is only going to evolve into more of a problem. In the next chapter, you will learn about how addiction comes to be. How did you become dependent on your addiction? There are many different paths that could have brought you here, and each one comes with its own baggage and differences.

GENERAL POINTS FOR REVIEW

- Addiction has been a problem for multiple eras and generations.
- These are the general signs of addiction: tolerance, lack of control, little to no interest in non-addiction related activities, affected social life, investment of energy on addiction, and withdrawal symptoms.
- Behavioral addiction and substance addiction are the two types of addiction.
- Behavioral addiction is the dependence on particular activities or behaviors.
- Substance addiction is a common type of addiction. It is the dependence on substances such as alcohol, and drugs.
- Addiction affects the brain, and in most cases, medication is the best treatment.

2

HOW ADDICTION HAPPENS

In the first few sections, you were given an in-depth discussion on addiction but you may be curious about how addiction manifests in your life or in the life of someone you know. How does it happen? How did you become this person who functions in such a way that you cannot live without using? People are not born with addictions, nor is someone with an addiction inherently a "bad person." The only situation in which babies are born with prior connection with drugs is when the mother used drugs while pregnant, and even in those circumstances it is not the fault of the child. The point is that there is a point where something indeed changes, and we will explore the different possible ways that alteration came about.

Addiction is not a two-step process, as we talked about before: you do not wake up, drink alcohol, and the next day, you are an alcoholic. Addiction happens over time, and usually only after consistent use of a substance or engagement in an activity. The path to addiction is slippery. One has to learn to draw the line between indulgence and overindulgence to avoid addiction. It is easy for things to get out of hand when you play video games for an hour a day, the next day you might want to play for two hours. The gradual increase could go on from there, and you could become addicted. Even this seems incredibly two dimensional, so we'll try another approach, one with a more personal viewpoint.

I smoked for years, decades actually. The first time I had a cigarette it made me light-headed and I felt nauseous, but my friends had been regular smokers for a few years and I didn't want to look completely foolish in front of them. Because of my incredibly low tolerance, and that I had come from a rather strict upbringing, I was firm about not becoming a "smoker." In my mind, there were several absolutes that separated a "smoker" from someone who casually and occasionally had a cigarette. One big red flag to me was buying a pack, sometimes a carton, and in my eyes that would end it all. Another was owning lighters and having an ashtray. It made sense in my mind that as long I knew the identifiers and maintained a distance from those identifiers, I could have my cake and eat it, too.

At that time, I was struggling with extreme stress and depression, my first real bout with these issues. I didn't drink and drugs were simply something to firmly say *NO* to, as I had learned throughout school. Cigarettes, however, fell somewhere in a gray area as far as I saw it. I was honestly looking for something to provide me with a distraction, not really an "escape" per say, but rather something to release that stress that seemed to have taken up residence in my chest. I didn't buy them so I would only smoke around my friends because I would ask my buddies for a cigarette when I wanted one - which still wasn't very often. My personal situation did not improve, though, and from that came more anxiety and more depression.

The change was so gradual that I didn't even notice it was happening, until one day I realized that I had a drawer with at least four lighters in it, plus two ashtrays. My justifications had been that even if I bent the rules on the outskirts of the risk factor - lighters and ashtrays - I could still avoid ruin by staying away from that core pitfall: buying a pack. You can tell where I am going with this, and within a few weeks I had my first purchased pack, heart crushed, but stress temporarily managed. I was a heavy smoker until very recently, and I still can't recall exactly how I went from getting light-headed to smoking several packs a day. Addiction is not quick, nor is it easy to track. This is something to keep in mind as you continue.

Many people go through rough times and some come out of the experience with scars - mental and physical - from trauma. Society, however, does not encourage people to address their trauma in order to move on with life. Boys and men, as a generalized gender in this case, are told to get over it; they are told to "act like men" so they bottle things up. Women and girls are dismissed as overly emotional. Neither of these cases is true, and both stereotypes are incredibly harmful to the healing process. The expectations on both genders to conduct themselves in a certain, preset manner despite outside events is ridiculous, and will have a lasting impact on a person. Male or female, the devastation caused by addiction is still a real, unbiased consequence.

Ignoring trauma does not make it go away. Instead, it makes the victim deal with the trauma in the worst way. While many victims of trauma end up hurting themselves or others through self-hate or violence, some turn to substance abuse or overindulge in habits and behaviors. While it is true that many aspects of our modern world are learning new, more efficient ways to treat addiction, there are still so many who are overlooked. Silence is never the answer, whether it is about getting yourself the help you need, or it is providing support to a loved one through their struggles. No one will make it through alone.

Many people use these substances and habits as coping mechanisms. They rarely have a plan in place to deal with their trauma. Instead, they usually aim to run away from it. Addiction, for many people, is a way to hide from pain and trauma; addiction is a tool for escape. It is easy to turn away from your problems, and even easier to depend on behaviors or substance use. The issue of dependency is a form of self-medication for many. It stems from the human tendency to run away from problems, rather than addressing and overcoming them. This is one of the reasons that addiction continues to thrive in society. If we were better at recognizing and then healing or dealing with our problems in healthier ways, maybe addiction would not be such a prominent issue in our society.

Addiction starts when your brain convinces you that you can not live without depending on a substance or habit. When you start taking a substance or engaging in activities that are potentially addictive, your brain encourages you to continue doing those things. As explained in the previous chapter, your brain releases dopamine when you engage in activities that it finds pleasurable. The brain releases this chemical when you hang out with friends, or read novels, or generally do things that are healthy and enjoyable to you, personally. Your brain does this to encourage you to do those things again; an incentive to live in a way that is conducive to overall health. However, when you continually use, your brain produces excess dopamine. This, in turn, causes your brain to reduce the production of dopamine - even though your body needs a certain level of dopamine to properly function. Your body makes up for the lack of dopamine by causing you to consistently use. At this point, a chemical switch occurs in our brain and we begin to depend on our addiction, believing that we need it to function.

Addiction is harmful to us physically and mentally but it can also affect those we love. Addiction drives people to do things they normally would not have done if they were not addicted. Oftentimes, people who are addicted sacrifice their love for themselves and others in pursuit of their vice. You may find that you lie to your partner about how you spend your money, or you may push your parents out of your life because they seem suspicious of your activities. Or maybe you borrowed some money from a friend to buy alcohol, and you know you hardly ever borrow money. It is through these seemingly little things that addiction begins to lead you astray.

This is why it is so important to maintain a stance of awareness when it comes to the subject of addiction and dependency. You know how you usually act, and you know what drives those actions. When something occurs that causes you to act outside of those usual parameters, it should be recognized and addressed. What happens instead is you ignore it the first time, or even the first few times it arises. You figure it was a rough day, or just an anomaly. It was nothing to take seriously, because when you stop and actually look the situation over, you are well aware of what you will find. By remaining in that place of awareness, you are able to notice when these out-of-personality changes occur, and recognize your patterns in order to stop the negative cycles or spirals before they take hold.

How does addiction begin to take over our lives? This hostile and destructive process usually starts from our biological side before it advances to our emotional side. Many people assume that addicts are people who lack self-control or are selfish, but research conducted in the last sixty years has proven that addiction has more to do with a person's biology than their will. It is easier to understand addiction when we realize that our human biology causes us to seek out things that are pleasurable to us. We can rise above our biology, however; this is where psychological, and societal factors come in. We are not slaves to our biology and that is why people can recover from addiction. This makes dependency similar to other diseases such as diabetes in that living a healthy lifestyle can help manage such afflictions. Research has shown that, like other diseases, some people are genetically predisposed to addiction.

While it is well known that the increase of dopamine upon constant use is what causes the "buzz" or reward that we chase after, recent research has shown another critical role dopamine plays in addiction. There are specific dopamine receptors that are responsible for the motivation to forgo instant gratification in order to work toward a greater reward. These dopamine receptors are also called D2 receptors and they are located in a region of the brain called the striatum. A lower dopamine response among D2 receptors can cause people to chase short-term rewards, and instant gratification – both of which are common behaviors in people with addiction disorders. Some people have fewer D2 receptors in their striatum, making them genetically predisposed to addiction. Those people with lower D2 receptors are more prone to impulsivity. On the other hand, there are people with higher D2 receptors who tend to be more successful in treating addiction from the perspective of behavior, i.e. through behavioral interventions. Some people have reduced D2 receptors not because they were born that way but as a result of constant use of substances or engagement in certain behaviors and activities that prompt a higher-than-normal release of dopamine. When the brain inevitably regulates the dopamine levels, the level of D2 receptors available in the striatum reduces, and those with addiction become even more likely to use and more impulsive.

The human brain, our mind, is a very complex organ. When our brains function properly, we are able to adapt to our environment with healthy coping mechanisms. It is this very adaptability of the brain that can have the potential to contribute to addiction. Having this affliction changes the brain's structures and its functions, as well as your ability to maintain a natural balance. Addiction also alters the brain's chemistry, causing damage that, in some cases, can be irreversible. Many of the symptoms associated with addiction are present as a result of these changes in the way your synapses are firing. For example, the brain's cerebral cortex is in charge of regulating potentially damaging behaviors such as compulsivity, impulsivity, and decision-making. When you constantly engage in pleasure-inducing activities such as drug use, gambling, or shopping, your cerebral cortex changes. This makes it less capable of preventing negative impulses, and you will have more difficulty resisting the urge to use.

The hypothalamus is a part of the brain that includes autonomic regulatory centers that regulate reactions such as stress. Substance use affects the hypothalamus' ability to regulate these reactions, causing people to use even more in order to relieve reactions such as stress, and fight-or-flight. When someone tries to withdraw from substance use, they are flooded with stress thus creating a vicious cycle. Another symptom of addiction that is caused by changes in the brain is the memories and cues associated with activities and the withdrawal symptoms that are triggered by discontinuing use. The brain's amygdala is associated with memories, cues, and emotion. The brain associates certain memories with certain cues, and any attempt to dissociate from such cues causes withdrawal. For example, if someone drinks alcohol every time they get home from work, the brain associates coming home from work as a cue to drink alcohol. This cue is stored alongside the positive memory associated with drinking alcohol. An attempt to stop drinking alcohol can cause withdrawal. The memory of withdrawal is unpleasant enough to serve as a powerful cue to continue the addictive behavior.

EMOTIONAL CONSEQUENCES OF ADDICTION

Addiction, over time, causes emotional instability in the life of someone struggling with addiction, and by extension causes instability in the lives of their loved ones. This type of mental disruption is dangerous because it can worsen a person's addiction and cause their lives to be taken over by their need to fulfill their dependent mind and body. It may not seem like it but people struggling with addiction often feel similar emotions with their loved ones. Loved ones of addicts often struggle with guilt and the feeling that they could have done more to prevent the addiction. Addicts often feel guilty about their addiction disorder, despite their inability to stop using.

The range of emotions linked with the entire process could stretch endlessly. It is because of the incredible complexity of the circumstances that the reactions of everyone involved run so high, both the reactions of the addict and the reactions of those who are trying to support them. It is not a low stakes situation, and will bring out depths of people that may not have been present previously. When something or someone people love is threatened, they will go to many extremes to ensure the safety of that subject. In this case it is how much those involved - including yourself - are going to let themselves be emotionally present.

Guilt

People who are addicted usually feel guilty for their behavior. For some people, they may experience guilt while using while others may experience guilt after using. During sober periods, or when they are done with the activity, they may experience guilt for the questionable behaviors they engaged in while using. They may feel guilty for making their loved ones suffer, whether physically, financially, or emotionally. Guilt is a dangerous emotion because the loved ones may attempt to make up for their guilt by enabling the addict. This will only worsen and complicate things.

This is one of the more driving forces behind many different aspects of the process. Guilt is a powerful emotion, a powerful force in general, and can either be a brilliantly positive catalyst or have an incredibly detrimental impact. The person who is dealing with an addiction most likely feels extensive guilt over what they are doing, but this does not always mean they will suddenly come to terms with what needs to be done. In fact, more often than not, people use this onset of guilt to shrink further into themselves, usually resulting in returning to the addiction - sometimes harder than before. This is why an approach that has guilt as a focus is rarely the right step to take. This "tough love" method can be useful in certain situations, but when improperly implemented, it can severely damage already harmed relationships and further affirm to the addict that their dependency is the only constant.

Helplessness

An addict may feel helpless because they do not know how to quit using. They may feel overwhelmed because they want to stop without help from anyone, but they cannot. Many addicts feel powerless and it is not uncommon for them to simply accept their situation. At the same time, the family and friends of an addict may feel like they are also helpless and unable to solve their loved one's afflictions to being dependent. Even though this group of people know that they did not cause the addiction, they know that they cannot control it either, and that does not make them feel any less helpless.

As with guilt, this can be a very powerful factor. There are few emotions as empty as *helplessness* feels. It can bring on a plethora of over-emotional forces - the aforementioned guilt, anger, self-loathing, to name a few - and the end result would be incredibly overwhelming. In truth, the only way to combat feeling helpless is to discover what *will* help. Usually the reason the loved ones feel this way is because they want to be the ones fixing the situation, the ones being there for the addicted party. Because they must rely on an outside source, or simply one that isn't them, they feel like they didn't assist whatsoever.

On the other side is the person struggling with their addiction. The feeling of helplessness is a constant already, and seeing the effect it has on their loved ones only increases that. Because of the destructive cycle they are in, their response to this situation is skewed. Rather than being able to think through the possible solutions, the mere idea of coming to terms with their issue brings on more isolation. From that comes more of the same cycle, thus producing more helpless moments.

Shame[1]

Shame is commonly felt by people struggling with addiction, as well as by their loved ones. This deep-rooted emotion can make a person feel less worthy than they actually are. It convinces us that we have less value than we do because of the situation we find ourselves in. This is how shame can eat away at an addict and those in their different circles. Because many people equate addiction with moral weakness or lack of self-control, people struggling with addiction, and those around them, can feel embarrassed to speak out.

Often the terms *shame* and *guilt* are used interchangeably, but they should be looked at and utilized separately. While both are very real and exist throughout the environments of addiction, they represent two very different emotions that originate from separate sources.

Guilt arises from feeling remorse, usually regarding an action you participated in or caused. This is a more internalized emotion, focused on what was done wrong and how *you* feel about it. The presence of guilt is not always a negative thing, and can actually be proof that you have sensitivity to the feelings of others.

Shame, however, is a much more painful, visceral feeling. Whereas guilt was about *what* you had done, the shame is due to the pain you caused *from* that action. It is an awareness that you conducted yourself improperly, and thus are going through a form of self punishment to mentally rectify the situation.

Both of these emotions regularly exist during the difficult process associated with addiction, but it is important to know the difference between the two and how they relate to ourselves, and the situation as a whole.

Sadness

Sadness is a very prevalent emotion in the life of an addict. People struggling with addiction may be sad about the opportunities they have missed out on because of their addiction. Or they may be sad about expectations they failed to meet. Their loved ones may be feeling this way because they witness how addiction limits the life of the person they care about. However it occurs, this should be an expected occurrence at some point - or many - throughout this process.

Feeling sad over something is a more reactionary emotion than an origin. For example, guilt and shame, respectively, may *bring on* feeling sad. You first must realize and understand that a situation is not what it could be, or that something is lacking, and then the sadness comes.

Fear

Fear is a very real part of the life of an addict and their loved ones. No matter how inconsequential or complex these fears are, they can negatively impact the decisions and thoughts of addicts and their loved ones. The extreme worries of addicts may revolve around their use – specifically where and when they can get their next fix. The similar feelings of the loved ones of addicts can range from fear of financial problems to broken relationships to incarceration or death.

A very dangerous situation can arise as time passes in regards to this fear. Each time you choose your addiction over a more positive option, you slowly wear down the voices of goodness and health that are trying to tell you otherwise. These, along with the other influences in your mind, are necessary to creating a positive method of living. Without fear, especially, you create a lifestyle where there is no consequence, no deterrent to the negative actions that are being done. Courage and bravery do not exist without fear, just as the ability to know where danger lies is also from having a healthy sense of fear.

It is very difficult to break free of addiction. For some people, once the negative spiral into addiction has been initiated, it becomes very difficult to get out of it. For many of the afflicted who struggle with substance abuse, it is very easy to lose that grip on reality. Constant use of alcohol or drugs can shorten the time an addict spends sober and free of the influence of their use. While it is more difficult for people who are addicted to behaviors to lose track of reality, it is not impossible. When a person spends hours on end cooped up in their room playing video games, they often lose track of reality. They may not know what time it is or even remember what they were going to do before they started playing. The same can apply to gamble addicts. They may gamble and lose track of time, or how much money they have spent.

Another way to look at it is that, for most people who struggle with addiction, there is nothing on the other side. While those who are trying to help them continue to reference how amazing it will be once sobriety is reached, and share success stories about a new, fresh life, this engagement is usually met with skepticism from the addicted party. Even the concept of a life free from the dependency is a distant dream, if it is still one at all. When those loved ones in the innermost circle speak of that "other side," the message falls on deaf ears. The miscommunication occurs because the addict does not want to stir up trouble, or endure the testimonials for much longer, so they respond in a positive, welcoming manner. This causes the supporting group to feel heard, and leave it alone for the time being, allowing the afflicted person more time away from the situation and finding solace in that escapism thought process.

It has to be real to them, the reward factor, and the promise. An addict makes ten thousand broken promises to themselves on a daily basis, so the idea of *something better* just over the horizon is a placation used to justify, rather than a reality of any sort. That is where the true challenge lies: how do you get that person to believe that there is something good, something better, waiting for them in sobriety. The unfortunate truth is that more often than not it takes the exact opposite. Rather than believing that something better was there, a painful rock bottom is reached, and from that comes the crossroads of a lifetime.

Oftentimes, addiction progresses from mere use or activity to the rationale for an action. When you start using cocaine because you do not think you can survive without it, or you need it to get through your day, you are truly addicted. The "birth" of addiction is when your logic is abandoned and your reason for an action is skewed in favor of your use. Addiction does not occur instantaneously; it is an accumulation of things that we have done over time. We often ignore these things or think them too innocuous so we charge ahead without healing from or reflecting on them. These things can be daily consumption of alcohol, or regular shopping, or even overly constant consumption of pornography and other sex-related content.

Everything in this process comes down to one key factor: awareness. Without awareness, you cannot hope to recognize the red flags or the opportunities for change. Without awareness you will not be able to see outside the haze of addiction. Without being aware, you cannot trust in those you love. Learn to trust beyond your perspective, and see through their eyes. It all starts with the ability to be mindful and aware. From that point forward there will certainly be challenges, but you will be prepared to face them with courage and resilience.

GENERAL POINTS FOR REVIEW

- Escapism and the refusal to address our problems can lead to addiction.
- Addiction begins to lead us astray when we dismiss our inhibitions to use, and we start feeling like we cannot survive without using.
- Addiction is not always a lack of self-control or will.
- Some people are genetically predisposed to addiction.
- Addiction causes changes to the brain's chemistry and these changes are the reason for many symptoms associated with addiction.
- Addiction emotionally affects addicts and their loved ones.
- Some emotions that are common between those struggling with addiction and their loved ones are fear, guilt, shame, etc.

3

UNDERSTANDING THE PAST IN ORDER TO BUILD A FUTURE

Addiction is a byproduct of unaddressed trauma and emotional pain. It manifests as a result of unaddressed and unresolved issues of the past. If you have financial issues that threaten to overwhelm you, you may choose to drink your way out of your problems rather than facing them head-on. Your financial issues are not going to disappear out of the blue. What happens is that you abandon addressing those issues for alcohol consumption which can lead to addiction. You need to understand and dissect your problems if you want to overcome addiction. The past is not to be run from, neither is it to be ignored and treated like it does not exist. But you should never dwell in the past. Dwelling in the past will most likely stunt your growth and progress. Far too many people get stuck fighting their past that they forget, or are incapable of, building their future.

Have you, since you decided to either begin the road to recovery, or to help a loved one on their path, examined the full origin of this particular addiction? I am sure that to one extent or another you have examined the factors that led to the various stages of your life, both in and out of the addiction cycle. Have you *truly*, from an almost academic viewpoint, stepped back and looked at the scope of your timeline?

Few people have, and that is because it requires increasing levels of honesty with yourself. You cannot have understanding, especially of your past, without the ability to be vulnerable and transparent. There are most likely some very serious issues that will present themselves through the events you have gone through, and without the permission to be that direct with yourself, it may end up just being a date and a label.

Your past is what it is. While that may seem simplistic, that is a good place to start. You can't alter your past, and even if you suddenly had no cravings, no hardships from the fallout, or any consequence to your life of addiction, you still wouldn't have erased or rewritten what has already been done. Too often this is misconstrued when people take on the path of recovery. They expect that somehow this new life of sobriety comes with a massive, time travelling eraser. You don't get that kind of a re-do, but you do get the chance to ensure the mistakes you made are turned into productive and positive results. *That* is the truth to hold onto. Set out to change your future, but do it from a position of learning from the past - not fighting it.

In order to overcome addiction, you need to find a balance between your past and your future. You need to properly, deeply, understand your past if you want to heal. If you simply forget about your past, you will not be able to rectify anything properly. The further you get into this process, you will find that your hindsight is not nearly as bleak. Whereas before you may have only looked back with shame or disgust, now you see the events that took place all had a part to play in forming who you are now. While you are probably not proud of those moments, you can find peace in knowing you are now taking those errors and relearning habits.

What does it mean to heal? Healing is overcoming and restoring oneself to wellness. True and honest healing purges you of the turmoil you went through in the past. It does not erase where you came from, but it makes things easy to bear. Finding a remedy is a byproduct of addressing the emotions and turmoil that you have been avoiding. It is important to know that with healing comes acceptance of oneself, of what is and has been.

The most powerful thing you can do on your journey to a life free of addiction is to resolve your past. Finding resolution to your past is to successfully accept that you do indeed have one, and understand that you deserve to move forward from it. The first step to take in resolving your past is acceptance.

ACCEPTANCE

Acceptance of oneself is key to true healing. What it means in this sense does not only refer to acknowledging your addiction and deciding that you cannot change; it means recognizing that you have issues and are addicted but you love yourself. In acceptance, loving yourself means you are going to do the best you can to become the best you can be. This begins with seeing the problems, and then formulating a plan knowing that you are going to overcome addiction.

Acceptance will change the way you see yourself and rid you of what is known as a "victim mentality." Victim mentality is a personality trait in which a person blames other people for the problems and challenges they face. People with this type of negative mentality do not own up to their faults, and they deflect responsibility for their actions from themselves to others. Oftentimes, people with victim mentality gain pleasure from being persecuted or pitied. Many people who struggle with addiction have a victim mentality. If you are such a person, you need to take responsibility for your addiction and cast off your victim mentality. When you do this, it becomes easier to free yourself of blame, as you free others of blame. All the resentment you feel toward yourself will drain away upon acceptance of who you are, and what you are going through.

This is a very difficult cycle to break as well, and you should not feel dismissive when it comes to the actual work involved. In order to maintain a life of addiction and dependency, there is at least a modicum of a victim's mentality required to justify the constant battle of self that goes on. While it is factual and known somewhere in your mind that you are not the victim in this scenario, you *have to* convince yourself of that in order to function. You cannot live in a state of refusal to give up your vice, maintain that you are the victim, and still claim stability without having that altered and skewed perspective. It is also for these very reasons that it is absolutely vital to not only fully recognize that pattern, but to reverse that thinking to properly see where either blame or responsibility truly lie.

FORGIVENESS

Forgiveness is the intentional process of letting go of one's feelings of anger, resentment, bitterness, and the need for vengeance toward someone who has hurt us, including ourselves. To be honest, especially in these situations, forgiveness most definitely includes ourselves. In some cases, forgiveness is more for you than it is for another person. Even in situations where someone offends or hurts you, forgiveness is a way for you to move on from that situation. Forgiving yourself allows you to let go of whatever guilt is weighing you down and delaying your journey to an addiction-free life. By forgiving yourself, you find gratitude and happiness even in the darkest of past times.

The ability to forgive is a character strength that more people should strive for. Some people are naturally more forgiving than others because of their personality but this should not deter you from improving your ability to forgive, especially if this is a trait that is difficult for you. People find it difficult to release themselves from that burden because they believe they do not deserve happiness. Other people may find it easy to forgive those who hurt them but are unable to forgive themselves for their past. It is because of all these factors that they may be unable to forgive themselves for their addiction because, as addicts, they believe they will relapse.

The key to moving on from addiction is to remember to always forgive yourself. Remember that your past happened and you cannot change it; what you can change is your future. You must choose to always forgive yourself for your past decisions if you want to move on to a healthier lifestyle. Forgiving yourself does not mean that you condone your past decisions, neither does it mean that you are excusing your actions in the past. It simply means that you have acknowledged your addiction, and you are ready to let go of the negative feelings and thoughts that you have toward yourself as a result of your past addiction. To properly forgive yourself, you have to accept your addiction. When this subject was studied, the results showed that forgiveness may sometimes involve grieving for what was lost. You may have lost your job, your family, or your finances. It is okay to accept what you lost because of your addiction and forgive yourself.

In my experience, when dealing with those who struggle with addiction, they are so hesitant to forgive themselves because they feel that not doing so is a form of penance. This is their way of making up for the time they wasted, the hurt they caused; in effect, it is a trade. They made a ruin of the time they were given, so now that they have found a life of sobriety - despite that, actually - they now must sacrifice peace to atone for the sins of their past. This is not only a severely incorrect way to view the situation, but it is also incredibly damaging. The entire point of emerging whole and new, after the harrowing experiences that brought you here, is to rediscover the inherent value that you possess. Among a list of other things, you gave up that value to yourself when you made damaging decisions after damaging decisions. The truth that you refuse to allow in is that it was *only to you* that your value had diminished. Public opinion be damned, because your worth never faltered and it is a heartbreaking situation indeed when the collateral damage to the choices you made ends up being the existence of any self-worth, esteem and pride.

Forgiveness is very beneficial to you and those you love. By forgiving yourself, you give yourself the go-ahead to mend your relationships that may have been damaged along the way because of your addiction. Forgiveness of oneself also encourages positive thinking, and it may provide you with a sense of hope for your future. When you no longer have a figurative cloud of self-hatred or disdain hanging over your head, you are more likely to see a positive way out of your addiction. While every aspect of this process for understanding is important, it all begins with the ability to forgive, to let that negative view of yourself become dim, and replaced with a triumphant, confident, absolved self image.

GRATITUDE

Gratitude is a feeling of thanks and appreciation for benefits received, and for life in general. One of the best things you can do for yourself is to express gratitude for the little things. For example, if you were addicted to a substance of some form, you can be grateful for the fact that you still have your life. Far too many people die from various overdoses of different substances. Gratitude is the key to inner peace. When you constantly express gratitude for even the littlest of things, the universe will send you more things to be grateful for.

When there is an element of dependency in your life, it is difficult to be truly thankful. The primary focus is survival, whether that is through avoiding consequences or the attaining of your addiction fulfillment. Only then are you grateful, and it is a fleeting moment, replaced quickly by a ticking clock for when you will need to survive all over again. You tend to experience relief more than actual gratitude, to be honest. That is another excellent reason why this particular aspect is one that has possibly been forgotten, or simply gone unused.

Gratitude makes you more positive and open to new opportunities and lifestyles which will be beneficial to you. Grateful feelings for how far you have come from your past to your present affects you and those around you. Your energy becomes more positive when you are grateful; it even tells on your environment. There is true joy in being able to feel truly grateful for what you have, rather than simply being content with making it to the end of the day.

Take a deep breath and look around right now. Take stock of what is around you and what it reminds you of. What reminder of gratitude stuck out to you first? Were there more than one? There is rarely a bad time to pause and remind yourself about everything you can be grateful for. In fact, it often provides you with that clear perspective all over again, a good way to reflect on the positive changes that have been made, and the people by your side throughout.

By resolving your past, you are telling yourself that it is okay to move on to greener pastures. It is okay to forgive yourself for your past and live a life free of addiction. It is okay to be grateful for the little changes that have had a positive effect on your life. When you accept your past, you bring yourself closer to a positive present, and away from the past. By being in the present, we deal with the truth of our reality. The present lets us know where we are in our progress, and we can assess ourselves to determine what we need to do to live better lives. In being present, we can make use of the numerous resources that are available for people struggling with various types of addiction. These resources aid in recovery from whatever addiction you struggle with. There are specific apps for people in recovery, most of which are free. These apps provide people with addiction treatment and resources for recovery. Because they are mobile apps, it becomes easier and more convenient to keep track of your recovery by monitoring your triggers, keeping a virtual journal, and connecting with people who are also on the journey to recovery from addiction.

Aside from mobile apps, there are more conventional resources that you can use. There are self-help groups and 12-step recovery groups that can be of great help to you and your journey to recovery. Also, there are government websites that you can consult to find qualified and accredited addiction treatment programs. Addiction-recovery organizations such as the American Lung Association and the United Kingdom's Institute of Alcohol Studies play crucial roles in your road to recovery.

One cannot move forward in life without having confronted one's past. Running away from your past without dealing with it would prove detrimental in the future. It may even cause you to relapse. It is dangerous to leave your past unaddressed as doing so would make it a permanent fixture that promises to darken your life at unpredictable times. You should also ensure that you do not remain in one position, even after your recovery. Having gone through acceptance, forgiveness, and gratitude, your next step is to redirect your focus toward building a new life.

The best way to ensure that you move forward in life is by taking things one at a time and doing things at your own pace. Do not rush into your new life, or think that you are doing worse than other people because they seem to have recovered faster and better than you have. It is your journey so you should not compare the steps you take to anyone else's journey. Ensure that you live – truly – and take each day one at a time.

GENERAL POINTS FOR REVIEW

- Addiction is a byproduct of unaddressed trauma and emotional pain.
- You need to properly, deeply understand your past if you want to heal.
- What does it mean to heal?

- Healing is overcoming and restoring oneself to wellness.
- Steps to resolving your past:
- Acceptance
- Rid yourself of the "victim mentality."
- It is vital to recognize your pattern.
- Reassess your thinking as to where blame is placed.
- Forgiveness
- Forgiving yourself is just as important as forgiving others.
- The ability to forgive is a character trait that more people should strive for.
- Forgiveness is beneficial to you and to those you love.
- Gratitude
- What reminder of gratitude sticks out to you in your life?
- By resolving your past, you are telling yourself it is okay to move on.
- One cannot move forward in life without having confronted one's past.

4

A BALANCED AND PURPOSEFUL LIFE IS A SOBER LIFE

Imagine this scenario: You have a stable life, comfortable finances, fulfilling relationships, and goals and hopes for the future. One day, through no fault of your own, you are in an accident of some sort. In the time following this accident, you had to attend physical rehabilitation and were put on a prescription to help manage the considerable pain the injury was causing you. Most nerve injuries have a tendency to linger when it comes to pain, and can be predominant even when the physical rehab is working.

You had never experienced trauma to this extent before, and considering the sudden halt to your normal routine, you feel off balance. Your stress levels began to drastically increase, and with that came the added difficulty of working through both the physical and emotional damage. As you continue with your recovery, you run out of your Paid Time Off, and quickly run through the remaining Vacation Time you have at your place of work. Your boss tries to be understanding, but after the lengthy time off he cannot hold your position any longer and you are let go from your job.

Now the stress rises exponentially as you must still continue to heal, but the challenges continue to mount. Throughout this time you have begun to discover that the only time you find a semblance of peace is when you are taking your pain medication. A shift occurs in your mind and rather than seeing that medication as a physical remedy, it is now a way to find solace from the rapidly deteriorating structure of your life. You find yourself using a few more pills than usual during the day, but you are still okay is what you tell yourself.

The financial burden continues as your insurance runs out now that you are out of work. You were smart with money so you have savings, but now you have gone through your first prescription, and you are increasingly aware of how many pills you have remaining, plus the refills you are being allowed. You haven't gone out as much, or nearly at all lately, and your friends have started to notice and are mentioning their concern.

Something in the back of your mind is aware that the way you are handling your medication is not healthy, but the thought of not having a respite from the stress causes those thoughts to be stifled quickly. More calls from your friends, more dodging and making excuses. It seems each time you do this avoidance dance with your social circle, you have to take more medication to mask the rising realization that you are on a dangerous path.

Fast forward another month. You are out of prescription refills and are painfully aware of how many pills are in the last bottle. You haven't answered the phone in three days other than to try and convince your doctor to cut you a break with another refill. You know that everything is crumbling, but as long as you don't have to see it, you are okay. Your savings will last another few months, but you are becoming more worried because you aren't as worried about the money as you are with the pill situation.

Another few months go by and you no longer recognize yourself. Every routine you had is gone and now replaced with a grim survival mode. Nothing is in balance, and each day is a dismal stretch of hours leading to sleep. You still aren't quite sure how you got here, but you know it isn't right.

This story is heard often about how easy it is for a life to unravel when imbalance goes unrecognized. While yes, the presence of medication and circumstance provided a welcoming environment for addiction, it truly takes hold when you begin to ignore the changes in priority around you. This chapter will cover the damages that living a life without balance can cause, as well as how important it is to be aware of these imbalances.

The choice to move forward in a life of sobriety is an incredibly hard decision to make, but what proves to be even more difficult is living a life of imbalance. In order to maintain a cycle of addiction, it becomes an absolute necessity to live a double life. Neither face is genuine and are both equally false. This lack of balance leads to the cornucopia of issues and deterrents to sobriety we had gone over in the previous chapters: anxiety, depression, and eventually a path towards even more back and forth between those two faces. Make no mistake, you have both the strength and fortitude to correct this imbalance, but it takes a committed combination of faith and time.

Take a moment and consider what areas of your life endured the most disruption due to your addiction? While most people see a general deterioration in areas of their life, there is usually a primary place where they are impacted in a somewhat disproportionate manner. It may be unpleasant to think back to those times and circumstances, but it is a necessary challenge. It is not enough to simply *know* there were areas of imbalance, you must identify to the best of your ability *what* those areas were.

Perhaps you became extremely isolated and that social hermitage began the chain reaction to the other aspects of your life. Or maybe you were able to keep a false stability across everything except for in your marriage, and subsequently all the fallout from the rest of your life was funneled into the dysfunction brought to that relationship.

The details will differ as you discover the specifics, but it is worth setting the book down for a few minutes and really thinking it over.

Just as the lack of balance creates disruptions throughout your life, having balance and maintaining that aspect of your routine leads to increased peace and an atmosphere that promotes healing. There is transparency in a life of balance, an open policy with yourself about where your focuses lie, and why you choose to prioritize as you do. Across the scope of your daily life, you have different obligations and desires for how your time is being spent, and with each choice, you create your priority list. By recognizing these moments, you will have a clearer picture of where your time goes, and if there are imbalances, they are there to be addressed.

If you find yourself at the gym more than anywhere else and your choices in other circles of life begin to rely solely on your working out, that is an indicator of a priority that may need a closer look. There is nothing wrong with having work be a priority unless issues arise that deeply affect your family and personal life. A focal point for you, something that seems singular, may be an indicator of a different way that balance can impact a life, especially when in or with addiction. Addressing this is not a moment of judgment, because even on days where things may seem to lean a certain way, it does not always mean there is an imbalance. The presentation of a new routine carved out by a singular focus on one part of your life, however, is where the scales begin to tip in a direction that could indicate an addiction.

By breaking aspects of life down into concrete, readable portions, it gives a chance to breathe and take in the information. Over the next few sections, you will be able to see different areas where singular priorities could have a negative impact on your life. When appropriately balanced and committed to positive change, these areas combined form a healthy, forward-progressing approach to living.

Health and Fitness [1] [2]

The path to sobriety runs hand-in-hand with maintaining a healthy lifestyle. The actions themselves are as essential as creating and having a schedule that provides structure. Exercise does not have to be complicated; simply, the presence of consistency will help form those positive habits. When going through the recovery process, some activities are correctly used to help build those foundations. These are VACI's, or Vitally Absorbing Creative Interests, as SMART Recovery defines them; exercising, crafts, nature watching, all of these are excellent examples that all aid in rediscovering what used to bring joy rather than merely replacing those activities - the type that got to the point where you had to be using to enjoy them, or that directly influenced your addiction.

Research has shown that it is just *doing* the activity that can bring benefits. Something as easy as walking for thirty minutes a day is beneficial. It isn't only the physical aspect of this that cultivates an atmosphere of healing and growth. By having pre-planned activities scheduled, you won't simply justify not going out, or not disrupting that. Simple self-talk can help, "If I have to get up and run in the morning, I can't go out tonight where I could get a drink." Other small statements of the same nature can assist in those moments of persuasion.

For many people, not just those who struggle with addiction, there has never really been an interest in exercising. Despite the fact that it is commonly known to positively impact practically every aspect of your life, we still distance ourselves from it. If you took an isolated route during your addiction, there is a good chance you did not have a dedicated exercise routine. The same can be said for those whose addiction made working out particularly difficult. The specifics of why aren't the point, but rather that it may require a shift in perspective. This may not be an interest you enjoy, per se, but rather one that is purely here to provide stability and longevity.

You have made it through truly monumental struggles that many have not been able to; that is no small feat. Keeping that at the forefront of your mind, you should have a desire to do everything in your power to keep this newfound life intact and functioning. You've earned this chance, and including a physical aspect will be beneficial in many ways you may have not considered. Some of those benefits include elevated mood, better sleep patterns, increased positive energy, a healthy distraction, lower stress, and improvement to your overall well being[3]. What others have you experienced or can you think of?

There are other aspects of exercise, not physical, that can be beneficial to the process. One common issue that those in recovery encounter is that they have much more free time than they had previously. Periods through the day or week filled by that addiction are now gaps of unscheduled, stagnant time. Adding exercise to the schedule is a catalyst more than merely a time-filler; the workout itself is rarely the focal point.

Depending on the type of addiction, your body has been put through various situations and endured more than it was intended to. Because of this, there are levels and variations of healing that must occur. While the physical portion of exercising may not always be the focus, it is a massive boost to that healing process. Balancing hormones that hadn't been released accordingly, increased nerve connections in the brain, and laying a foundation for a more balanced sleep schedule stem from the physical healing gleaned during working out.

The world of exercise is expansive and sometimes complex for someone who has never really delved into that realm. To avoid disruption to your momentum, or any doubt in yourself, here are some examples of recommended workout routines specifically for those in recovery[4]:

- **Walking**: Especially early on in your recovery, you may not have a lot of energy. Withdrawals are also especially tiring, so this can be a good use of your time as well as getting some form of physical exercise in. Never discount the benefits of a brisk, thirty minute stroll.

- **Hiking:** This could be a gentle step up from the walking routine. Aim for the environment rather than the physical exertion. Being out in nature for extended periods of time has proven to have a plethora of benefits, ranging from physical to emotional. If you are an enthusiast, then feel free to go full pace with your equipment and effort but you should feel no obligation to do anything other than a mildly challenging, nature-based walk.
- **Yoga:** You would be hard pressed to find a group that discounted the positive effects of doing yoga. From increased breathing awareness to flexibility, the opportunities for bettering yourself can all have a firm anchor in the calm that yoga can bring. The varieties are growing every day, and thanks to its recent popularity, it is easy to find a local center that hosts classes. If the social aspect is intimidating, YouTube has an excellent library to choose from, all from the comfort and non-judgemental eyes of your own home.
- **Swimming**: While this may not always be the most convenient form of exercise, there is no denying the overall workout obtained from a mere twenty minutes in the pool. The main benefit is that it is a very low impact exercise, in case soreness or aches are particularly bad that day. As with the other exercises and suggestions in this section, you should feel no obligation to join a class or even do anything in an organized manner. Having the water around you and just floating can be exactly what you need.
- **Dancing:** Here is one of the more unorthodox suggestions, because it is often overlooked. A reason that people choose this over other forms of exercise is because it doesn't really *feel* like you are working out. There is an inherent aspect of fun that may not always be present in other methods you

have tried, or were considering. Another incentive is that many dance studios offer a first class for free, or at least a trial bargain. This has the potential to be a low-risk, fun, healthy, and social activity to give a try!
- **Team Sports:** While not as simple to be a part of, this may be a more relatable form of working out for those who had some sports influence in their life. Again, there are many variations of activity, along with different levels of skill and experience. You should never feel like you are overextending yourself with the addition of exercise, and when considering an organized team sport this should be a point of thought.

Team sports could also be an avenue to discovering something new! While the popular sports are well known, maybe do a little research and find a sport you never really gave consideration to before. Curling, badminton, or cricket are just a few examples of some less common variations you could try. You never know until you give it a shot.

- **Weight Lifting:** Finally, this is a more structured, typical approach to working out. While it is common and most gyms or workout rooms tend to have some form of weights, proceed with caution. Unless you are under supervision or have prior training, do not push yourself when it comes to weight training. While the basic act is simple, the potential for injury by taking on too much is a risk that you need to be aware of.

With these examples, hopefully you now have a better idea of ways to incorporate exercise into your schedule as a regular occurrence.

Spirituality[5]

Every person differs in their belief systems and how they view the concept of a higher power. Regardless of the differences between religions, the ability to turn to something larger than themselves plays a significant role in gaining and maintaining stability and balance. No matter the specifics of what you believe, there is a consistency when it comes to finding the power within. That place inside yourself, somewhere to turn to in daily meditation, is a healthy step in learning *how* to heal, and not only allowing it to happen.

The basis of spirituality is faith. Not only religion but faith in yourself, that circumstances can change, that belief in hope. Cultivating this creates a nurturing environment for a positive self-image to take root. So often in recovery, there is negativity in every version of self one can have, and this becomes both exhausting and deteriorates that gleam of hope.

Where exercise can impact mental health and is completed through action, faith has the ability to heal both the mind and body. The belief that there is value in who you are as a person is an invaluable characteristic to build, and this is begun deep within yourself. Where this aspect applies during the recovery process is a personal journey, but never forget that your strength of spirit can and will bring healing.

In a recent study by Adi Jaffe, PhD[6], he broke down the approach to spirituality while in recovery as being between two main camps of thought when it came to this subject. It was the Religious group and the Spiritual group, and while both have positive messages and can be essential for certain people to their success in recovery, both are vastly different.

Those from the Religious group tend to recognize a deity in some form, usually in a structure or order. The people who subscribe to this belief consider it necessary to commune in fellowship with those of a similar system and ideologies. This is where the Spiritual group differs. Having spiritual qualities does not directly infer the presence of a greater being, but is more of an unseen connection among all of us, a cosmic understanding and bond, of sorts.

While there are obvious differences between the two, they can converge on several key aspects in a healthy life free from dependency. Both schools of thought have variations of focus on returning a purpose to your life. They also believe in being a contributing member of society and the world - the order differs depending on the specifics. Along with these, the overarching idea that both camps agree on is finding something greater than yourself to believe in and use as a basis for faith.

Religion finds that in a god, or multiple gods, whereas Spirituality focuses on the belief that by coming together as a society, the best of ourselves, that real change can be affected; both within ourselves, and for the world.

Social Life[7]

During a discussion with a friend some time ago, the cutting of ties while in recovery came up. It is a commonly accepted truth that with the admittance of addiction and the subsequent recovery process, there will be a circle of friends with whom you will no longer socialize. This is usually considered one of the hardest steps to finding healing and peace through recovery. There would be unconditional acceptance across the board in an ideal world, and minimal changes would need to occur if any. Sadly that is not the case. As common as that is, it is just as common for that social gap to remain unaddressed.

There may arise the need to replace friends or that fewer friends directly correlate to lessened value. You lose no value when you choose your health over specific friends because while you cannot change the choices they make, you can distance yourself from a potentially toxic environment. This is not an easy decision but you must understand the power within it. You are giving yourself back the power in your life, and there are truths that go with attaining a healthy balance in your social realms.

One aspect that is certainly a truth and yet is rarely considered during the process is that things *will* change. While there may be some people you associate with that will be accepting of your choices and direction in life, many will not react how you may have expected at all. If you are not prepared for this then any balance across the other components of your life runs a risk of becoming unstable.

Do not discount the importance of this aspect. As we explained at the beginning of this chapter, isolation is an extreme detriment to your well being. This is one of the earlier red flags to be aware of, but it is also important to keep in mind as you are now rebuilding both yourself and your life. Yes, there may be relationships and areas that simply cannot be fully repaired, but you knew that real life consequences would occur. What you *can* do is find resolve to use that mistake, as with the others in your past, as a catalyst, an inspiration, to always be better; to always move forward.

Romantic Life[8][9]

Within recovery, it is commonly known that the maintenance of yourself and your sobriety is fragile in the early days, and could continue to be well into the process. It is because of that fragility that dating and any romantic endeavors are put out of mind until one year has passed. This alone can be a subject of contention and has been debated from multiple views over the decades, but what benefits to balance are there from waiting?

First, understand that this period of waiting is not any reflection of value or saying that you shouldn't have rewards from the new life of sobriety. This a moment you have worked hard for so, of course, you should be able to fully experience this fresh side of life. By not giving this the proper respect, because your sobriety is a serious matter, there is a risk that either priorities or perspectives could be skewed. It all comes back to balance and this particular subject is one that has more of a tendency than most to create that imbalance.

It is a natural characteristic within humanity to steer in the direction where the heart directs. It is a driving, strong force, one that begins to increase when a relationship begins to form. That type of connection brings with it a mass of complications that are difficult to maneuver in any circumstance, let alone for one beginning to learn balance within recovery. The desire to please and fulfill one's partner can be a powerful pressure to backslide into common patterns. It isn't merely the possible experiences while in a relationship, there is a real chance for disruption to your balance if these relationships end.

Throughout this process there will undoubtedly be times when you feel judged, attacked, pointed out, or that all the guidelines and expectations are unrealistic. Every one of those concerns is valid and should be considered extensively during your recovery. Relationships and romance can be a great boon or a disastrous journey no matter your past. Just like you had to admit your addiction, you must come to terms with what the recovery process is like and what future disruptions could occur.

Your health and your sobriety are always a singular focus. Find balance within that and romance, and all the ups and downs that go with it, shall come in time.

Hobbies

While in recovery there are two types of hobbies that you can undertake: productive ones and those for leisure. These two can intersect for certain activities, but most that you choose will fall under one of those two categories. Both are crucial to the process as they provide stimulation and are an excellent use of your "swap time," or time you used to devote to recovering from your addiction.

Hobbies are an excellent use of time, and they provide necessary distractions to curb the cravings. There is no need to feel pressured into picking up hobbies you have no interest in simply to *have* them. Taking enjoyment in the activities you choose is crucial to maintaining that overall balance in your life. One of the first, and most important steps you took on this journey was admitting the addiction, and with that comes the acceptance that the road *will* be difficult, that cravings will happen. The structure of these hobbies is a healthy way to alleviate the weight of those times, in addition to creating that foundation of stability.

Just as we discussed with exercise and working out in general, your skill level has nothing to do with the activity or hobby. You may not be training for the Olympics, but your effort and time spent will result in benefits to both your health and path of sobriety.

Career

This can be a touchy subject for certain people depending mainly on how your addiction impacted your work. Some addicts maintained a stable work life and let the imbalances fall to the other sectors of their lives; many others saw a direct and negative effect at their place of work and on the quality overall. It is precisely because of these reasons, and that is a trigger subject, that it must be addressed.

No matter the program you are in for recovery, there is a section or step regarding work and careers. It is a part of life in general to not only seek out work, but to find one that fulfills and rewards. That does not change due to your recovery, in fact you may find that your work life has *more* meaning. As with your personal life, you had to either hide or work your addiction into your routine to avoid being found out. This is an exhausting cycle and the burden alone brings with it anxiety, stress, and directly impacts your performance on the job. Stepping forward in this new, refreshed life will feel new and situations that had brought paranoia or triggered your addiction can now be stepping stones and reminders of the changes you have made, and are continuing to make.

A career can also be an excellent goal to work towards. Depending on your past, furthering yourself at work may not have been an option due to either substances or time needed for your secrets. A brand new road is before you now, and with that comes increased advancement opportunities if you stay the course. When those difficult moments arise you will have a concrete reason to push through without giving in!

Be prepared for the moments that trigger your addiction, especially in the workplace. In a perfect world, the transition would be easy and every situation would be ideal without the hint of temptation, but you know full well this will not be the case. Even under the best of circumstances you will still encounter those moments from time to time, but that does not reduce their importance. You are going to have more time on your hands and you will be aware of these times. When a cigarette smoker decides to quit they will no longer take smoke breaks. Suddenly they are painfully aware of the 5-10 minute periods they used to have, particularly if those breaks were based on a schedule. A coworker in a previous job told me that, for him, the hardest times were thirty to forty-five minutes after he got to work, and after meals. By identifying those specific times to expect the cravings to hit he gave himself the chance to be prepared. Applying these methods to your workplace is telling yourself that you have value, enough to put thought into things of this nature.

While every aspect of balance we covered can be individually applied to your journey, they are all moving you towards a bigger picture. Early in your sobriety these are used to create a foundation, something to build from towards your brighter future. These experimentations of pursuits are moving pieces that navigate you to your purpose. That is what it all boils down to: what will your impact on this world be?

Your life has both meaning and purpose. Addiction caused a temporary disruption of your road towards that goal, but it in no way destroyed it. Patience is key in this process, and by allowing every step and progression to arrive in its own time you are allowing yourself the vulnerability to accept it when you are ready. Outside of yourself there is no one who can tell you your calling, but when it happens it will feel right.

Don't fight this feeling when it occurs. Sometimes our past can make us hesitant to accept rewards or positivity because there is a part that feels we do not deserve it. That somehow by sacrificing good things we can help make up for mistakes and negative actions committed. This is a misguided reaction, though a very relatable sentiment. You will be working to uphold your sobriety for the rest of your life, you do not need to cause yourself grief to satisfy guilt. Instead, find closure and solace in the joy from furthering this new life you fought to regain.

Discovering your purpose has little to do with you and more to do with the effect you will have going forward; that is precisely how you know it is your purpose. A selfless instinct takes over and it is about the work, bettering humanity and everything around us. It is important to remember this because too often we are searching so hard that we search right past our path. There is a fluidity to this process; a flexibility to let things happen and move forward in the steps you know to follow. Everything starts somewhere, and keeping these guidelines in mind will give you direction when things get tough - and they will, but you are tougher. Much tougher.

Your past is exactly that and is behind you now. The issues have been addressed and you are in a forward motion. Part of this is accepting that your present is allowed to be rewarding and success is something you are deserving of. Living with an intentional balance and in a purpose-driven way makes sobriety a pretty straight forward path. This is not to say that it isn't fraught with obstacles, but with the keys you have learned the path forward is clearer.

Regarding these obstacles you have been given a checklist of your own design as we've moved through this chapter. The aspects of balance - *Health and Fitness, Spirituality, Social Life, Romantic Life, Hobbies,* and *Career* - provide something to reflect back upon if you recognize a pattern emerging that could lead to relapse, even early signs. Going through your balance keys will give you a better view of what is causing this disruption to your progress. There is no room for judgement here, in fact you should be praised for putting effort into ensuring your success in a sober life. Losing balance creates that sense of instability that can trigger an episode of engaging in vices.

You have value and worth. From that you are worthy of patience, from others and from yourself. Everything learned here is put in place for the benefit of anyone who is willing to commit not just to a new life, but a balanced approach to that lifestyle. It is with all this in mind that the next part of the journey begins. Patience is needed throughout the balancing process, as it is needed when you begin forming new, healthy habits. This is what we will cover in the next chapter.

GENERAL POINTS FOR REVIEW

- The lack of balance leads to a cornucopia of issues and deterrents to sobriety.
- What areas of your life endured the most disruption due to your addiction?
- By breaking down aspects of life, it gives a chance to take in the information.
- Keys to Balance:
- Health and Fitness
- Walking
- Hiking
- Yoga
- Swimming
- Dancing
- Team Sports
- Weight Lifting
- Spirituality

- Social Life
- Romantic Life
- Hobbies
- Career
- Your life has both meaning and purpose.
- Going through your Keys to Balance will give you a better view of what is causing disruptions to your progress.

5

DEVELOPING NEW HABITS

The life of one in recovery is a life of habits, whether these habits brought you to your addiction or those that you are forming now to heal from those decisions. As you no doubt know, some habits form easily and smoothly fit into our lives. Others, more commonly, take dedication and time to build up.

Now that you have begun to reverse those old, destructive habits, you can move forward in confidence towards starting new ones. Everything has an origin, and the creation of these positive new habits begins with simple, daily choices. This is going to be a slow process, one that will require small steps, truly walking before you run. In no way is this a race and haste will not serve you well on this journey. Take comfort in this fact. It is a rare thing indeed in this life to have a reason to slow down and think, plan, and *then* act. Depending on your type of addiction you may have experienced the pace much faster than you were comfortable with; this is a gift, not just the opportunity that recovery presents, but that you have the time to take this at a healthy, steady pace.

There are several reasons that defy common sense showing that forming these new, positive habits are beneficial to the new leaf you are turning over. As discussed previously, having time on your hands during this phase in your life is certainly inadvisable, if not directly harmful, and you know that this free time is an inevitability as a side effect of your sobriety. These habits take that time and put it to a good use; thirty days to build a habit, we've heard this, and that is one month that you will be putting time and effort into this work.

Take a moment to think about what habits that you either have or are planning to begin as part of healthy routines. Just as the process of creating habits takes time, so does the process as a whole. Allowing yourself the freedom to pause and absorb when needed is going to be crucial to avoid feeling overwhelmed.

A large part of recovery is understanding that you are not alone with the struggle, not alone with the urges, and certainly not alone with the human weaknesses we all must battle. It is in these times that being self-aware becomes important. Without that awareness, the feeling of being alone can evolve into something much more dangerous to your health and well being. Going from feeling alone to a spiral is too close a connection to risk over simply not noticing. Being here, fighting to regain your life, signifies that you are *much* stronger than that.

Along with being aware of letting feelings become a road to regression, it is vital to be aware of old patterns that could emerge during times of difficulty. Before recovery, your usual reaction to an obstacle or hardship was to turn to your addiction, or at the very least begin conducting yourself in ways that will lead directly to it. Recognizing the formation of these old, negative habits will go a long way towards avoiding them.

A good definition for these negative habits is *a patterned behavior regarded as detrimental to one's physical or mental health*[1]. The key word there is "pattern," and for those in recovery, this can be a trigger word but it is certainly relatable. Just understanding that it *may* happen is not enough, you must identify what brings about those cycles of destruction. There are many variables that come into account when discussing the catalysts for these patterns, so let's look over a few[2].

- **Observance can be key**. Notice changes in yourself, or your surroundings, that reflect behaviors leading to or directly correlating with your addiction.
- **Expecting immediate perfection**. Keep in mind that recovery aims to progress you to a place of peace and healing, not a fast track to a result.
- **Keeping old perspectives**. Even though you have made significant changes in your life, especially concerning your addiction, you may still have ways of thinking that became so common they are now instinct. "More is better," could be one, or "try anything once." The wording isn't the point, but rather the possibility of that thought process's destination.
- **Recovery in a rut**. Just as recovery is not a quick fix, there is no maximum timeline either. How long you are in the stages of recovery vary greatly from person to person. Feeling stuck or stagnant can be a path back towards old patterns.

These are just a few possible instances to be aware of. Perhaps you didn't relate to any of these. That is okay, and it gives you the opportunity to use your self awareness. Ask yourself what your variables are that could lead back to old patterns? It doesn't have to be a direct action or traumatic event, but rather, as in the list above, it could be a perspective shift or a thought process.

Just as the negative patterns and cycles of behavior can lead back to the life of addiction you left behind, there are positive reciprocals of those same patterns. By implementing these in your life you allow yourself the benefits that come from sober, healthy routines. These can be across a broad spectrum, and it is important to give yourself time to discover which ones work for you. If you got no joy whatsoever from flying kites, it most likely will not make for a good hobby. Not that it isn't a healthy, outdoor activity, but rather that you will give you no emotional benefit, and tension caused from not enjoying it can turn the situation into a negative experience.

You deserve to have hobbies and routines that you take pleasure in, as long as you recognize the responsibility you also have to your sobriety. So instead of kites, maybe you prefer watching documentaries, or playing chess. Whatever you end up deciding on, remember that you are not relegated to a single hobby. Keeping an open mind and an attitude of awareness will be a large help in this discovery of enjoyment.

There are aspects of this process that are rarely brought up for the public view. If your addiction involved a substance, no doubt it enhanced special activities or made mundane ones enjoyable. Perhaps your addiction itself was the enjoyable activity, or one that brought you the feeling you desired: overeating, self-harm, and the like. However you came across it, once you remove yourself from the addiction, you may find that activities lack interest of any kind. This is normal and with effort and time will begin to be rectified. Your body and mind had become used to relying on the chemical release from the addiction for the euphoric feeling, rather than an activity bringing it about in the intended biological fashion. So now you must retrain both your body *and* mind in how to release those chemicals correctly. You are fully capable and empowered to achieve this, and excel while doing it! Patience, effort, and you make the unbeatable team that has already come so far. Imagine how far you can go!

Take a moment to think about what positive habits you have picked up since you started this new, fresh journey. There is a very good chance that you have put something healthy into motion without even realizing you were establishing a new pattern. Here are some possible options that you could consider, or maybe to add to those that you already are doing:

- **Cleaning.** Chores around the house, dusting, polishing can be both productive and healthy. If repetition is a positive tool for you, consider this as a good habit replacement.
- **Communication.** Isolation is a massive red flag, and has probably been an aspect of your life during your addiction. By reaching out more often than you used to, you allow for transparency to be cultivated. Family and friends, especially those who are familiar with your struggles, are excellent sources for support. A fun conversation is always a boost, as well.
- **Find peace.** Being mindful is a key factor in your journey. "Mindfulness is the basic human ability to be fully present, aware of where we are and what we're doing..."[3] Adjoining this mindset with the practice of meditation creates an atmosphere of growth, healing, and honesty with yourself. All of this translates to a better sense of self, better peace of mind, and a healthier step towards the life you are trying to create.
- **Exercising.** As we discussed before, do not be intimidated by the word *exercise*. You are not being asked to train for the Olympics - to train for anything, actually. Rather, it is the act itself, as minimal or intense as desired, that creates the new, healthy habits. Getting yourself into the pattern of being active in some way is an important variable of recovery. Do not be afraid to look for that one thing that piques your interest; yoga, Crossfit, or even just jogging a little. It all works, and it will all benefit you and your sober lifestyle!
- **Learn something new.** Depending on the places your addiction took you, there may have been many conversations at the peaks of the highs where elaborate plans were made to do such and such, and when the slope of the crash hit no actions were taken. This time is different, because *you* are different. Finding a new skill and putting the time and effort into learning it can be both satisfying and incredibly

therapeutic. The possibilities are vast, so take your pick with your triggers in mind.
- **Books or podcasts.** Both of these can be fruitful. Another factor to consider is attention span. If yours is particularly low, maybe try an audiobook rather than a physical book. You can still get the story, or the impact of the words, but you don't have to be singularly focused on it, which can often trigger anxiety and spirals if not handled correctly. The same goes with podcasts. Perhaps newspapers or magazines are not matching with your preferences, but you still want to have an intake of news and entertainment, or any subject you desire. By searching for and listening to a variety of podcasts, you will be taking positive action, but without stress and tension.
- **Cooking.** You are not aiming to become a Michelin-rated chef. This is about finding an interest that can help form new habits. By learning new recipes and techniques, you open yourself up to healthy avenues for your energy.
- **Diet.** This can go hand-in-hand with the cooking habit. By taking an active interest in your well being - and this includes the physical aspect, as well - you place value on yourself. Don't be afraid to try something new here, because you never know what could end up being an unexpected favorite!

All of this may seem like a great deal of information, and that is because it is. Starting fresh, especially in recovery, means retooling yourself for a world that you have most likely been avoiding for years. Simply because you feel overwhelmed does in no way mean you are underprepared. Expect to feel the struggle, but do not expect to give in to it.

Depending on the route you have taken, you may have had guidelines or suggestions made to you that require what could be considered "deleting" old habits and replacing them. It is important to not feel pressured into completely removing portions of yourself. The reasons you became addicted are usually directly linked to characteristics you possess. There is a tendency to steer yourself towards what interests you, or what could possibly enhance those interests. This does not simply mean making cartoons funnier or getting through long shifts without needing sleep, it also pertains to a desire for numbness, or to detach. These are interests as well, and you cannot discount their impact on how you make connections to activities or hobbies.

The reason that being asked to completely discard these connections seems so daunting is that the achievement is virtually impossible. This is not an issue of replacement, but rather of using that same energy and mindset to redirect your activities and time. Everything is done in steps, and this process is no different. Jumping in before preparation is taken into account will rarely result in something beneficial. Rather, begin by creating a space for these redirected patterns. This can be within your schedule or an actual, physical space in which to cultivate. Effort translates into increasing the value you recognize in an action. Because you are taking the time to create stability rather than rush to an immediate goal you are giving these new tools and what you have learned the chance to take root. Focus on each footstep along the way, not the destination you are heading towards.

It is important to remember that there are many different roads you can take on this fresh start to your life. There is no singular method, no sole process that leads to a sober utopia. Instead it is a matter of utilizing your self awareness and being mindful, quiet, and vulnerable in the present. One of these possible processes is a training technique called Habit Reversal Training[4].

This is a series of steps that help identify habits through awareness, and how to act in a more positive and healthy manner moving forward. You could consider this a form of impulse control, or a way to address damaging, consistent behavior. While we are going to unravel this process and break down the sections, remember that actually undergoing this type of therapy and intervention is done under observation and the responsibility of a trained professional. Not only that, but the conditions were closely monitored as well, ensuring that health and safety were the primary focus.

If this seems like something that will work for you, allow yourself the openness to unbiasedly view the series of actions and steps that make up this form of habit adjustment.

The actual implementation of the Habit Reversal Training is done by first Gaining Awareness, then Developing a Competing Response, Relaxation Training, Building Motivation, and finally Generalization. Every step is interconnected with the program as a whole; if, however, you find pieces and phrases that speak to you, hold those close and remember them. Simply because you cannot conduct this type of therapy on yourself does not mean you cannot gain something from learning about the applications.

Gaining Awareness

Without self awareness, you cannot hope to have a consistent, healthy, and sober life. By recognizing "destructive patterns," you are better prepared to identify them as they arise.

Developing a Competing Response

This is a rewording of a very specific form of replacing one habit with another. These can be large, sweeping adjustments, or small, detail-oriented changes.

Relaxation Training

Some people refer to the process of altering habits like this as a form of "self surgery." It isn't pretty, it usually hurts, but it is for your own good in the end. Because of this you *must* expect the struggles of anxiety, stress, and pushback from your own mind as you progress through this. Learning to relax and ease off the pressure will be vital in maintaining your will and energy throughout this process. By being able to have that relaxation ability, if a trigger presents itself you can respond in a healthy, calm manner.

Building Motivation

In this step, there is a combination of response techniques used to influence how motivation is utilized. Both negative and positive reinforcements are put into use to create balance. The positive aspect could be praise from those aware of your struggle and the process, while the negative could be the judgements you still see from people who haven't been able to forgive or let go yet. Both satisfy different aspects of the program and work together to help the formation of new habits.

Generalization

As the final step, this is where you learn how to transfer what you have learned into a real life setting. There is a major difference between learning a process and putting it into implementation. The responses you will get, and the reactions, will be guidelines to how the process is going and where adjustments may be needed.

This technique has been through trial-and-error studies since the 1970's, always under the consistent eye of both psychologists and neuroscientists. It is important to keep coming back to this point because the steps and process laid out in this book are for self-help, and while the topic of Habit Reversal has been covered, it is still a professional method.

Part of the process of creating these healthy habits is learning how to incorporate them into your routine. As a first step when out of recovery, the routine stands as a paramount aspect of this entire journey. Many times when those in your position go about trying to find interests to productively use their time, or simply to distract themselves from those cravings and pangs of addiction-related nostalgia, these attempts are met with obstacles. While "new" elicits a picture of something fresh and open, it can become problematic when looking at it from the perspective of assimilating this into your schedule.

Consider a change in perspective first, and putting things into practice second. Instead of seeing the new habits and your current routine as two separate entities that have to be somehow combined, look through a positive lens. Your routine is a functioning, changing creature, not a concrete, unmoving tablet of rules. As you learn and adjust to a sober life, your priorities will shift and the way you conduct yourself, and your time, will change accordingly. It is precisely because of these characteristics that introducing a new habit into your schedule is an organic process. There is no end-all method for doing this, and as such you must allow for trial-and-error. See where these new activities or interests of yours line up with how you allocate your time and go from there.

With this in mind, let's move forward into different ways you can incorporate the examples of positive habits we covered. Keep in mind the fluidity of your schedule and that you should be striving for flexibility, these pointers can help.

- Pick a time to wake up every morning that is conducive to your schedule, and stick to it. Use alarms or your partner helping or whatever can be a positive motivator to wake up at that time every day.
- Ensure time in your schedule for exercise. If you leave it to "when it happens" you are not cultivating structure.
- Meal planning can be a good, repetitive use of time that has productive results. This can work well into the cooking and diet aspects we covered before.
- Your well-being extends outside your mind and your physical self is a large part of it. Establish a self care routine that can help that same structure, but also one that will establish value within yourself.
- Household cleaning can be tedious, but when viewed from

the perspective of personal growth, it becomes a productive use of time. Consider creating a Chore Schedule to help put those habits into practice.
- A big part of self-care is hygiene. Depending on what path brought you here, that aspect may have suffered in the past. Seeing yourself as a person of value, and therefore worth the effort, is revelation in action.
- Finally, developing new skills is not only productive, it continues that trend of self worth. You may have lived from day to day in a survival mode, as many in recovery have. The future extended only for as long as the high, rush, or numbing lasted. Then everything was focused on continuing that feeling. You are on a different road now, a road of compassion and love towards yourself. By learning new things, big or small, you are telling yourself that there is a future to be worked towards. A future you want to be a part of.

These are guidelines and if you do not feel they mesh well into the sober lifestyle you are cultivating, then there is no harm in reading them and moving past. If, however, you feel a defensive reaction to any of these, then take a moment and explore that. Why would your first instinct be to go on the defensive? Maybe it was simply a knee jerk reaction relating to a past experience, and if so that can be addressed in itself. If the reason is because you feel attacked, that can be a signifier of something that needs exploratory if not invasive "self surgery." You are making these changes and implementing these actions for the betterment of your life and everyone you interact with. You can give yourself that few seconds to find the origin of your instinctual reaction.

You have been given a great deal of knowledge in this chapter alone, but the most important habit, one of positivity and progression, is that of Gratitude Reflection. This can take many forms - journaling, verbal pep talks, mindful focus - but the core principle is to create an atmosphere of gratitude and recognizing the moments that deserve that attention.

Journaling can be a key aspect of this and one that has the ability to keep the positive momentum going. Acknowledging these moments of thankfulness is not always enough. Our daily life is filled with interactions, conversations, thoughts, media, and countless other things that fill our minds. To expect that, on a daily basis, you can think back over the course of your day and pick out those key times when you noticed the need to be grateful is not realistic. Those are not just passing moments that get a nod, they are important and they matter much more than you may think. Keeping a journal doesn't have to be a line by line review of your day, nor does it have to be some ultra-personal confidante for secrets and whispers. It can simply be a Gratitude Journal. Its sole purpose is to document when these little bits of thankfulness crept in, and how often. That will provide you with a scrapbook of sorts to chart your journey.

Were there weeks where the pages seem a little blank? Or, on the other side, perhaps you notice a pattern where you had an overflow of these moments. By identifying them you can understand your reactions more, and see the world for the wondrous place it is.

Now, there are those of us who never took to keeping a journal. The reasons are not the important part, what *is* important is that not having that outlet creates the same issue as thinking you'll remember those significant moments. If journaling itself is not appealing, consider taking up meditation or schedule a daily, quiet, isolated time for yourself to reflect back on the day's events. Whatever the method, the importance is in the recognition of those moments of Gratitude Reflection.

The BAART Program (Bay Area Addiction Research and Treatment) has been serving the city and area of San Francisco since the 1970's[5]. From their expertise and knowledge came many different techniques and methods by which to treat many addictions, primarily those with an opioid history. Among these were five habits that would be foundational in creating stability within a sober life. Some of these touch on aspects we have covered, so the focus will be more generalized.

1. Eat a Healthy Diet
2. Add Exercise to Your Schedule
3. Practice Healthy Sleep Habits
4. Form Connections With Others
5. Nurture Your Interests[6]

As you can see, many of the programs and resources devoted to helping those who have chosen a sober path have similar bases in thinking. While ideologies and how to implement certain practices cause differences among these various programs and organizations, the fact remains that with the focus on your well being, your sobriety, and your future, you will have no trouble learning strength and how to continue your forward progress.

It is a mantra worth having: small steps, small steps. If you prefer quotes, then, "Rome wasn't built in a day." Regardless of the presentation, the truth remains the same. You are a person of value, and through that perspective, you can change the habits that were detrimental and build up positive, new habits that will encourage you to flourish. With patience and the correct view of your self worth, nothing is beyond your reach, especially stability and happiness in a future that is safe and healthy.

You are capable, you are strong. Never let those words slip your mind.

GENERAL POINTS FOR REVIEW

- The life of one in recovery is a life of habits.
- Now that you have begun to reverse old, destructive habits

you can move forward in confidence.
- A negative habit is *a patterned behavior regarded as detrimental to one's physical or mental health.*
- What brings about your cycles of destruction?
- Observance can be key
- Expecting immediate perfection
- Keeping old perspectives
- Recovery in a rut
- Just as there are negative habits, there are positive, productive ones
- Possible healthy habits to consider:
- Cleaning
- Communication
- Find peace
- Exercising
- Learn something new
- Books or podcasts
- Cooking
- Diet
- Habit Reversal Therapy:
- Gaining awareness
- Developing a competent response
- Relaxation training
- Building motivation
- Generalization
- Have you tried journaling as an outlet/positive habit?
- Five foundational habits for creating stability (BAART Program):
- Eat a healthy diet
- Add exercise to your schedule
- Practice healthy sleep habits
- Form connections with others
- Nurture your interests
- "Rome wasn't built in a day."

6

STAYING ACTIVE TO MOVE FORWARD

Change is never easy; this you know very well, and we've covered how change can take a variety of forms. There is a saying, "The best revenge is a life well lived." This is applicable because a common reason that those in recovery struggle in finding fulfillment in their lives post-addiction is that they feel they need to be punished for what occurred. Every time they falter or stumble in their journey, it is seen as an inevitable consequence of living the way they had been. This is a myth that *must* be dispelled immediately. Your past is what it is, and the way you rectify the wrongs and ripples caused by it is between yourself, your sponsor, and your loved ones. Make no mistake, you do not deserve to punish yourself. What you *do* deserve is to cultivate a life that will give power to your sobriety. You deserve joy and success and this can only be done by first finding forgiveness from yourself.

This concept is difficult for those who have not experienced life in recovery. When work is put forth and rewards are given like promotions, bonuses, etc., it is very common for the sober employee or friend to feel they are not worthy of this recognition. The logic is that somehow, over time, the amount of times you sacrifice the chance for something good, you get closer to a moral balance. Do you find it hard to accept praise? If you have been promoted since you began your sober life, did you feel like you couldn't accept it or that you didn't deserve it? These are not uncommon reactions, and by utilizing your self-awareness, you can be more cognizant of when these situations occur. It takes willpower and strength to put those kind of instinctual reactions aside, it isn't easy, but you are fully capable of accomplishing this!

Once you are able to not only see yourself in a future, but have that future be one of success and positivity, you have taken a large step. The key term is *forward*. Stagnancy, as we've discussed, rarely breeds progress. Just as the steps you've taken up to now have put a focus on seeing value in yourself, seeing a future for yourself creates worth as well.

While you may struggle with aspects from your past for some time - which is normal, and should be expected - understand that it holds no power or sway in your life now. You will always associate certain thoughts or even lessons with things in your past, be it good or bad, but it is not a place you can dwell. There is a method sometimes used when handling extreme trauma in a time-sensitive situation: letting emotions in. What that means is to allow yourself a moment to truly feel what your mind and soul are experiencing be it grief, joy, guilt, or the other countless feelings you could have. You only allow it to exist for that moment, though. You are in control. This technique can also be used when you experience those feelings that make a healthy future seem out of reach or not deserved. These reactions are a direct result of guilt, and while they are not a true reflection of who you are now, they exist and are real. Because of this, but for only a few moments, feel it. Understand the depth of the emotion, and then take back control. This will not be easy the first time, or even over the course of time, but the repetition creates the signifier of importance. You have placed value on this and will therefore put in the necessary effort to attain it.

When it comes to control, has your past caused you to place limitations on your present self? This goes back to feeling the need to punish yourself for your past actions. Your present is something fresh and new that's not controlled by your past. Do not allow the stigma that has been placed on those in recovery to taint how you view your future. There is a judgement that can follow those who struggle with addiction, and it is not only incorrect but also damaging to the progress trying to be made.

You've explored new interests and allowed yourself to be vulnerable, and all of it is done in pursuit of creating a balanced life. It all comes back to balance, and remembering to keep yourself in check regarding this. Refer back to the list of aspects in your life that require attention, and how they are prioritized. When you feel "off" or like you may slip, take stock of how the balance in your life is. If you are truly honest with yourself, there is most likely some part of your life that isn't being given the priority it deserves. Life is life. That sounds redundant but, at the end of the day, it's a simple truth. No matter if you are in recovery, an athlete, a lawyer, unemployed, or any other walk of life, life is just that: *life*. Expect turbulence, expect the road to become cracked and difficult to traverse, expect to stumble. Once you accept those facts, you can be ready when they occur and prepared to correct any imbalance.

It requires humility to take those steps, and you have developed the tools to put that humility into practice. By moving forward with this attitude, you can be vulnerable in the face of a world that is harsh and unfeeling more often than not. Do not be disheartened in those moments, because it is very easy to be overwhelmed when your skin is thin. There is an inherent fragility that comes from a person being open and vulnerable; the knowledge is that such vulnerability may cause them harm, sometimes deep and lasting. Your well-being is well worth that effort, and as long as *you* are dedicated to both the process and the belief in yourself, the risk will result in reward.

Action. Nothing happens without it, and in its absence there is detriment and imbalance. There is a very good chance that at some point in your past you tried the "wait and see" technique of avoiding consequence and responsibility. If you were a student of this body of thought then you also know the results are negative, and usually to a much greater proportion than if you had taken action. You know the story well, I'll bet. Someone runs out of means to feed their addiction, so they engage in something illicit or illegal to obtain the resources. Once they are able to use, the fear of being without fades and any future consequence also drifts away in justifications. You knew full well that the wrong action you took to get you the substance or means will have a reciprocal response, and the longer it goes unaddressed, the greater the consequence grows exponentially. By the time the high wears away or the numbness melts to feeling again, you are left with a stark realization of what it took to get you there. You weren't ready to address the underlying addiction and undergo the necessary changes, and the only action you can think to take is no action whatsoever. If you wait, then at least you have the time until you're "found out" to enjoy calm.

From that point, everything begins to snowball. No doubt you have to act in more secrecy than usual because you assume everyone knows what you did. Still you remain silent, stoic, waiting it out. Early in your addiction, you most likely got away without consequence a few times and that created a sense of being untouchable, so you saw it as a viable option when faced with a crisis stemming from your addiction. Inaction followed by more of the same eventually creates an ugly, distorted result where the hurt is spread over multiple parties and the damage is sometimes beyond what even you imagined. Everything comes back to one thing: the decision not to act.

Your life did not magically turn itself around and start on a new, healthy path. It wasn't an accident; you did this. You made a conscious decision to take action, going against every instinct you had built during your addiction. This same ideology applies through the remainder of your journey. Every day, you have to make that choice all over again. Routine, as we covered earlier, is a critical part of a balanced life, and including that choice into your schedule makes it all the more real. Say it loudly, repeat it as many times as you need to because when your health, future, and well being are at stake, there isn't room for feeling silly or judged. Never accept anything less from yourself than the courage that brought you here. Take action every time, especially when it seems like the most difficult thing to do.

Your life is a byproduct of the actions you take. The mistakes in your past are linked to a lack of action as equally as the times you decided to continue in your addiction. Creating an environment where you can string together a series of positive actions will continue that healthy cultivation of self you have been striving for. Keep it in the back of your mind, the forefront, and on the tip of your tongue at all times. *Take action!* Take action for yourself, for those you love who support you, and because your future is worth it. *You* are worth it.

Just as inaction can be detrimental to your success in a sober life, a lack of goals will also impact how you progress towards the future. Earlier it was explained how in your past you lived without a future; survival was the singular focus and anything else was trivial. The difference is that now survival depends on your positive choices rather than in enabling an addiction.

When you look ahead in life, far down the road, what do you see? Have you considered it? How far ahead do your plans go? Maybe you have a 5-year plan, or maybe you are still learning how to expand your thinking from a day-to-day agenda to something with longevity. However you are going about it, the point is to have your eyes set on goals, both short- and long-term. This is not only to ensure you are prepared for what is to come, but also because stagnancy takes many forms. A lack of vision for the future is often overlooked.

When those in recovery recount experiences, some of the keywords used are *haze* or *blur*. That is the entire point, really, in feeding that addiction. When the concept of time becomes based on a series of highs and lows it will feel chaotic, unkempt, and out of your control. The point is that you gave up your control of your own time to your addiction, and now is the time to take it back.

Why is having goals so imperative to this process? To living a healthy, sober life? It gives you back ownership of your time. You can schedule and plan weeks, months, and even years to attain the goals you set before you. Don't hesitate to make multiple variations as well. Have specific short term goals, have those that you wish to accomplish within 5-10 years, and then give yourself the freedom to imagine the apex of your success. Where is that place for you? By identifying that dream, that goal, you give power to it. It is no longer just a quiet desire in your mind; it is alive on paper or in text in front of you. Keep this list of goals close to you, no matter how short or long your list is. Folded in your pocket, written on your phone or computer, the medium isn't the point. The point is simply having it on hand as a reminder in difficult moments. Don't be afraid to look it over whenever you feel unbalanced or off your usual routine. Give yourself back ownership of time that is truly *yours*.

When the idea of time comes up, you must also prepare yourself for when your addiction tries to regain control of you and ownership of your time with it. It isn't a violent grab either, this you know all too well. It is a gentle coaxing, a caressing and reassurance that this is the right way to go. That you "deserve to feel good." In response to that in particular, you *do* deserve to feel good and on *your* own terms, not the addiction's terms. Until you find that balanced point and understand the awareness of self needed, then implement it in your life, you have to be ready for when those gaps in your time give way to those creeping thoughts. In those moments, the early time on this journey is when you will build the foundation that your future can be built on. It is a base of personal strength, willpower, and taking back control over both your goals and your time.

Once you view your future as attainable, and understand how to own your time, you can make the push forward towards that unfolding life. You are not simply going through the motions of recovery, your goals are real and are *yours*. You must come at this from the perspective that your goals and the steps to them are not solely part of a plan to prevent a relapse. There is a much bigger, much more important picture going on and it has you at the center.

Throughout this journey you have been building towards the goal of a well balanced, healthy, sober life. In order to achieve this, a plan has been formulating, created from the guidelines and lessons you have picked up along the way. It is vital to have that plan, that preparedness, when you are working towards the future you desire. That includes benchmarks as you reach certain points in this growth.

As with any program designed to enhance your personal growth, the two main types of goals are broken down into short- and long-term. Both are important to the final result, just as they are equally substantial towards maintaining. People learn and are rewarded in different ways, and the attention to that individuality means being aware of how you respond as well. Do you know in what way you are best rewarded to stay motivated?

Are you long-term oriented? Primarily focused on what will happen down the road, and the larger, more time-intense goals act as a motivator? People who have these tendencies are less inclined to see the more immediate, small-reward goals as a catalyst; they instead see these short-term goals as more of a distraction, or even an inconvenience. If this sounds like you, gear your sights towards those larger, big picture destinations; trying to force a system on yourself that is not efficient for you has no benefits.

Now, maybe you are motivated by those short-term goals, and that is perfectly fine as well. Without knowing your individual preferences and what best propels you forward, you will not be getting the most out of the processes you undertake. Focus on the smaller goals, the "stepping stone" goals. You won't be cannon-balled out of the water by the concrete results, but the practical applications and how they make you feel will be more fulfilling than if you made yourself wait for a reward that made the journey there less impactful.

Your well being and health are at stake, so ignore all those outside voices and listen to your own self: what form of learning speaks to you? How will you be motivated best to stay the course? *Those* are the real, important questions to be asking. Luckily, the answers are just as important.

A significant term was used previously, and used often, throughout this book. That word is *guideline*. The reason that this specific expression is used is that you should always refer to experts when it comes to concrete, practical advice. While every technique and lesson has been created to better serve your sobriety and teach you how to best prepare for the long haul of a healthy, refreshed life, it is not medically certified. In short, this is **NOT** a replacement for a prevention plan, any support groups, doctors, or any other form of professional help that you have been getting, or need to obtain. Now, it is an excellent resource and guide during the time you are in programs, or during any point in your new, sober life. What this plan **is** at its core is about bringing the life of your dreams to reality, while maintaining your well-being and health.

Keeping that in mind, the next chapter will show you how to combine the lessons you learned in Chapters Four and Five, and also how to review your progress without judgement. You are strong, empowered to succeed, and your efforts will get you there!

GENERAL POINTS FOR REVIEW

- Change is never easy.

- You deserve joy and success. This can only be achieved by forgiving yourself.
- Stagnancy rarely breeds progress.
- Feel and understand the depths of your emotions then take back control.
- Has your past self caused you to place limitations on your present self?
- Action: nothing happens without it, and in its absence there is detriment and imbalance.
- Avoid the cycle of secrecy.
- Your life is a byproduct of the actions you take.
- When you look ahead in life, what do you see?
- How far ahead do your plans go?
- Five years?
- Day by day?
- Having goals gives you back ownership of your time.
- You are building towards a goal: a well balanced, healthy, sober life.

7

IN REVIEW

Do you remember the different aspects of balance we covered? This Spectrum of Balance will come into play quite often as you navigate the sometimes choppy waters of sobriety. Let's take another look across the different variables that play a role in how balanced a life you are leading. As you make your way through the Spectrum, again, it's to review one of the core principles to the maintenance of your healthy direction. Whereas before you may have skimmed the cover, now we'll reopen the "book" and give a more intense look at the Spectrum of Balance and its varied and moving parts.

As we re-explore these different components, do not be afraid to put your thoughts and answers onto paper or document them somewhere. It is important to be able to chart the differences and improvements starting with when you first began your journey. It is important to see balance as both a priority and a necessary tool that will help you in maintaining sobriety.

A very important rule to keep in mind when going through times of review and reflection is to do it without judgement. This may seem like it should go without saying, but self-judgement and guilt are far too prevalent in the life of those in recovery. When you and others on the same path were feeding the addiction, you rarely allowed yourself the chance to feel the brunt of the emotions from the consequences. Once the haze and numbness are gone and you feel the full weight of the fallout, it is far too easy to live a life of self-hatred and derogatory actions. If you are in that vein of thinking, any nostalgia is tainted with a lens of judgement and undue rage. This mindset does not promote growth; more importantly, this mindset can start to erode the progress made up to that point.

As we continue onward, you will be asked to look back at and reflect on the progress you've made. You may feel triggered by this. Prepare yourself and actively withhold being overly harsh with yourself. Do not be afraid to remove yourself from the situation momentarily in order to reestablish an uplifting environment. Always make time for this when you feel it is needed.

Health and Fitness

This is one of the more important VACI's (Vitally Absorbing Creative Interests) because it not only takes time, it also directly correlates to several other elements of the Spectrum. When you first read through the section in Chapter Four, did anything about your lifestyle then stick out to you? What methods or routines have you put into place since then? Remember that no matter how often, or for how long, you exercise, simply putting the effort to working it into your schedule has created that attention to balance.

Spirituality

As this section in Chapter Four explained, the issue of faith and spirituality will differ from person to person, as will the role it will play in your sober life. In the time from then to now, how have your beliefs or faith impacted how you go about your life? Remember that this element does not specifically relate to religion, and in fact can exist without any integration - now or ever - to any creed. Having faith, especially when recovery is involved, is more about believing in *yourself*.

Take some time now and considera few things, either in your mind or on paper. How did you feel when you first addressed this issue when it was brought up in Chapter Four? No matter the positive or negative feelings related to that moment, it is important to recall. Now, consider where your faith is in your progress, your life, and your choices. Has it strengthened? If so, where have you seen the most growth. In what circles of your life has it made an impact?

All these questions, and any more that arise during the time taken to give it thought, will enable you to take a step back and view the larger picture. Without belief in the path you are on, without belief in yourself, you cannot be fully set up for success in a life of recovery.

Social Life

Too often this subject matter is put in a negative light when it comes up in review, or at best is viewed with sad nostalgia. While the unfortunate truth, as we discussed earlier, means that ties had to be cut socially when you decided to enter recovery, that is rarely unavoidable. It does not, however, define your entire social identity, especially now as you continue to progress and grow as a person.

Rather than thinking back over what you lost, consider it from a different perspective. What people comprise your support system? It is worth the time to write their names down. By doing this you are putting power behind your gratitude and recognizing those who helped you get to where you are through their efforts and belief. Look through the list you just made and really *see* the people you accounted for. In what ways did they positively impact your journey on an individual, personal level?

Your path here has taken social sacrifices, and those sacrifices were meaningful to you and as such will leave an imprint. During your time from then to now, and truly your recovery as a whole, you have no doubt let your mind think of those you had to distance yourself from. It is for this reason that you are replacing those feelings of nostalgia with the positive power of naming your support group.

Keep that list close and in times when you are lacking confidence or the road seems particularly rough, you can remember that you are loved. The concept of "being loved" can often seem off-hand and emotionless without an anchor in reality, and seeing the names of people in text is proof that this love isn't just an idea, it's a reality.

Romantic Life

Depending on where you are in your recovery, you may or may not be in a place where you are considering adding a romantic element to your life. Programs differ, as do personal preferences, so make sure that is all taken into account when this subject matter is brought up. There is never a rush to form romantic attachments, nor should there be any pressure. As you know by now, any rush will create an imbalance and is not worth jeopardizing your sobriety.

Where are you at this point? If you are still leading up to a point where you will allow yourself that chance, what plan do you have in mind for handling that situation? There should be an expectation of difficulty. Not just in the relationship, but in how it relates to your recovery. The road of recovery is one that lasts for the remainder of your life, as you know, and a romantic interest will impact and be impacted by your life.

On the other hand, you may be well into your sobriety and romance is already incorporated and an important aspect of your life. If this is the case, how does it affect your day-to-day experience? Whether you are in a relationship or not, including the possibility for both attraction and involvement, your sobriety will and must play a role. You lead a life of transparency, and in that spirit any partner you consider including in your life needs to be allowed the chance to consider how it will impact *their* lives as well.

Write out how you view romance, either out loud or on paper to give it power and how you've acted on it. Look at this from three different stages: when you began your sobriety journey; when we discussed it first in Chapter 4; and where you are now. This will let you examine how you've grown, and how your views of romance have either changed or remained steadfast. Love is a vital component of life, and will be a part of yours in some way. Without being able to see how this aspect has been viewed on your journey, you cannot appreciate it and be prepared to take on the responsibility.

Hobbies

While this element of balance can seem simple, it is just as important as the other aspects. Stagnant time is the enemy of sobriety, and as we learned earlier, simply *having* a hobby gives you an outlet when faced with time that has the potential to be unused. When you began this book, did you have any particular hobbies you had taken an interest in? Do you still participate in them, and if not, why did that end? Sometimes activities and other interests are in our life only for a short time, and then they have served their purpose. This is not a negative way to conduct both yourself and how you use your time. Allow yourself the freedom to alter what you put your time and effort into. Your life is centered around your sobriety, and from that will come a great relearning of various habits and patterns. Without the flexibility to adjust along with those changes, you will create unneeded friction in a process that is challenging as it is without any help.

What new activities are a part of your life now? Big or small, it is simply their presence that can matter. If you stopped some hobbies, take a look at why that happened and how you grew from them. As you review these areas, take the time to see how these hobbies and interests impact your schedule. Sometimes you may not realize you are spread too thin until you see it laid out in front of you. If you haven't felt stressed from these activities, chances are you have planned the time well, but it is always worth checking on. Consider it a form of allowing for self-correcting.

Career

The decision to begin a life of sobriety has had an impact across all areas of your life, but there are often more severe or direct consequences in several key areas. Your family and friends are one, and another primary element is how your work, your career, has been, and will be, affected.

Imagine that you had to make a progress chart that showed your job performance. You would plot key moments during your addiction, immediately following your decision of recovery, up until it was directly referenced in Chapter Four, and then now. How would that line's movements look? Where are the peaks and low points? If you feel so inclined, go ahead and sketch out a graph like this. See if you can really think back and calculate the ups and downs so they're plotted into an image. Make it as simple or as detailed as you would like; the goal is to give you a good idea of the progress as a whole.

Once you have done this, and hopefully have had a little "art class" fun while doing it, let's examine the results. Look at the particularly high points; to what real life events do they correlate? Do the same with the areas that are at the lowest. What patterns do you see? How have you made progress within those segments of time laid out before? Perhaps you will notice that you actually need to examine why there isn't more upward movement to where you are now.

The point is to take stock of where you may need to make adjustments, or perhaps to show that you are making the correct steps to ensure your sober life continues. Career can be where you suffered most because of your addiction, and can be the most difficult area to remedy as one in recovery. Do not feel discouraged, regardless of what you find in review; you are making great strides, and the benefits will pay off in their own time.

This may have been the first time you did an in-depth check on how the full spectrum of balance was holding up. Like anything that is a priority, it requires attention and maintenance as time goes on. None of the decisions and practices you are putting into action are single-use, end-all solutions. They are methods and steps along the way. It is important to go back and do these kinds of reviews to ensure you are living a balanced life, because in the hectic, fast-paced world we all must exist in, it can be far too easy to lose track of where the imbalance may be.

Keep the notes and points you made during this self-check so whenever you go through the Spectrum in the future you can refer back. There is a difference between *knowing* you are making progress, and *seeing* the progress you are making. Keeping this kind of information on paper or electronically will prove invaluable later on. Having a visible record will help you create goals and desires to work towards, with concrete reasoning behind them.

Every lesson and guideline you have learned and implemented during this process has all been for a singular goal: to create a balanced system to cultivate your sober life. Every piece is a necessary component to form a lifestyle that is designed to not miss out on any of the richness you can experience. This approach can be referred to as the "never a dull moment" method, or more simply, ways to keep yourself busy, but sober.[1]

A commonly agreed upon truth is that free time is rarely a positive element to occur during the sober routine. This is not saying that your immediate response to having that time will be rushing back to the addiction, but it *does* open the door for thoughts that could very well lead down that road. Until you are more grounded and have proven over time - to yourself and to your life - that you are able to handle those quiet moments, you are susceptible to unhealthy patterns of thought. Guilty ruminations and "what if's" can let doubt seep in, undoing the great work you've done on your confidence and willpower. While it may seem like a harmless event, it is not worth the risk to allow that kind of thinking to take hold.

New habits are difficult to implement, and for the first 30-60 days is a fragile thing indeed. Nearly everything you put into place when starting out on a path of sobriety *is a new habit*. Everything is going to begin from a very fragile place, and will need an added modicum of protection. This protection comes in the form of "time usage." While it is true that there are times when simply "keeping busy" won't be enough, but for the odd times when those empty slots do occur, you'll know how to react.

This process can be a slippery slope to navigate, because while you try to avoid those free times, it is also a necessity to include rest and downtime for yourself. Early on it can be a fine line between the two, and the process should be treated with focus and respect. Where are those places in your life that sparked difficulty early in your journey? How did you respond? Always being on guard and at the ready can be tiring, but it is a necessary challenge for that time. It is for these reasons that having a support system - and leaning on them when needed - is absolutely crucial to succeeding in this new lifestyle.

How are you making time for rest *and* ensuring that time isn't simply empty space that your mind can fill with unnecessary thoughts? This answer will be different for everyone, depending on situations and schedules, but the foundation needs to remain the same: doing everything actively and with awareness. That is how you navigate those sometimes murky waters of knowing when to let go and rest, and when to recognize the time as a negative atmosphere, and responding accordingly.

Maintaining a sober lifestyle is a never-ending pursuit. Day-to-day efforts and beyond, it is a challenge, but remember that it is a challenge you are certainly up for! Aim for success and sobriety and you will be able to follow through with the tools and methods you have learned here. Never stop moving forward with determination and a focus on your goals. Your addiction will always be waiting for you to come back, so you must remain actively aware for the sake of your health and well being. You are *worthwhile* and from that you can find the strength and purpose to persevere when the days seem too long, or the stresses are taking their toll.

Remain steadfast in your avoidance of boredom or idle time that could lead back down paths of negativity and destructive tendencies. You have worked too hard for these emotional pitfalls to ensnare you; take strength and courage from the tools provided in these lessons. You have a purpose, one that you may have lost sight of for a time, but now on this new, fresh road, you can set your sights back on those destinations.

Because of the work you do every day without fail, you have created the framework that can be utilized from here on out. You are empowered to say *no* when you feel a situation will not serve your best interests. The sacrifices made to form a healthy environment will give you the backbone, the power, to make those difficult decisions. Nothing is impossible when your mind and body are working in harmony. Nothing is impossible when you are moving forward towards a brighter horizon with patience and grace. The troubles of your past can be left behind for good and you can feel the freedom to progress in a life without limitations.

You are capable!

You are strong!

You will find your way to lift the weight of addiction.

GENERAL POINTS FOR REVIEW

- Do you remember the Spectrum of Balance?

- As we re-explore these aspects, are you recording your thoughts somewhere?
- Journaling?
- Digitally?
- Voice recording?
- Health and Fitness
- What changes have you made?
- What habits have you put into place?
- Spirituality
- How has belief impacted your life and sobriety?
- This is not necessarily religious belief, but rather a belief in *yourself*
- Social Life
- Whose names are on your list of supporters?
- In what ways did those individuals positively impact your journey?
- You are loved.
- Romantic Life
- Where are you at this point?
- What plans do you have for handling this aspect?
- How does it/will it affect your day to day life?
- Are you living a life of transparency?
- Hobbies
- What hobbies did you have when you began this journey?
- What hobbies do you have now?
- In what forms are they helping you self-correct?
- Career
- What does your progress chart look like?
- Did this give you an idea about your progress as a whole?
- What patterns did you notice?
- Have you made progress in those areas?
- Free time is rarely a positive element to introduce to a sober routine.

- Nearly everything you put into place when starting out on a path of sobriety is a *new habit*.
- Where are the places in your life that sparked difficulty early in your journey?
- How did you respond?
- How are you making time for rest?
- You are empowered to say *NO* when you feel a situation will not serve your best interests.
- *YOU* are capable!
- *YOU* are strong!
- *YOU* will find a way to lift the weight of addiction.

8

CONCLUSION

In this book, you learned how to balance your life, what triggers to identify, and how to live a sober life without judgement. You were challenged and asked to unearth depths of yourself that had been locked up for years, possibly longer. From the beginning, it was stated that by following the steps and lessons along the way you would find purpose, discover new positive characteristics about yourself, and how to live a life free from the weight of addiction. Standing where you are now, I have no doubt you are the living proof of all those elements!

There are few things in this life as difficult as finding the resolve and strength to battle your way out of addiction's grasp. Like many before you, and the many that will follow, you have accomplished something truly incredible. At one point, or several, there may have been no hope, no light, and no love. Yet now, in a new place, you are well on your way to being back in the brightness of sobriety: with hope, in the light, and truly loved.

Here is where our paths part, but in no way are you ever alone. Look to those you love in times when your strength doesn't feel like it's enough. Look inside yourself and find belief in the amazing places you will go and the incredible things you have yet to do! There are not enough words to define the bravery in a life saved by recovery. No one understands that bravery better than you do. You should be very proud of yourself, and every single day from here on out, you deserve to be reminded of that fact.

Thank yourself for this opportunity, and I also thank you for having the power to take control of your life. Addiction is one of the most difficult things in this world to overcome, and you have done that and so much more! Keep taking each step with power and confidence, because you are a being of joy, truth, and strength. Never forget that.

Thank you.

REFERENCES

1. WHAT IS ADDICTION?

1. https://www.verywellmind.com/willpower-101-the-psychology-of-self-control-2795041
2. https://www.ncbi.nlm.nih.gov/pmc/articles/PMC5068365/
3. https://www.ncbi.nlm.nih.gov/pmc/articles/PMC5068365/#ref-39

2. HOW ADDICTION HAPPENS

1. https://www.psychologytoday.com/us/blog/shame/201305/the-difference-between-guilt-and-shame

4. A BALANCED AND PURPOSEFUL LIFE IS A SOBER LIFE

1. https://www.smartrecovery.org/vaci-3/
2. https://www.smartrecovery.org/benefits-of-exercise-in-addiction-recovery/
3. https://castlecraig.co.uk/blog/2019/05/07/7-best-exercises-for-addiction-recovery
4. https://castlecraig.co.uk/blog/2019/05/07/7-best-exercises-for-addiction-recovery
5. https://www.rtor.org/2019/08/12/sobriety-spirituality-and-mental-health/
6. https://www.psychologytoday.com/us/blog/all-about-addiction/201805/7-spiritual-elements-critical-addiction-recovery
7. https://www.hipsobriety.com/home/2014/11/11/sobriety-your-social-life-the-8-things-i-wish-i-had-known
8. https://www.evergreendrugrehab.com/blog/love-sex-and-relationships-in-recovery/
9. https://www.ashwoodrecovery.com/blog/guide-to-relationships-after-addiction/

5. DEVELOPING NEW HABITS

1. https://alcoholrehab.com/addiction-recovery/bad-habits-in-recovery/
2. https://alcoholrehab.com/addiction-recovery/bad-habits-in-recovery/
3. https://www.mindful.org/meditation/mindfulness-getting-started/
4. https://www.floridarehab.com/treatment/addiction-therapies/habit-reversal-therapy/

5. https://baartprograms.com/about-baart/
6. https://baartprograms.com/5-healthy-living-habits-during-recovery/

7. IN REVIEW

1. https://lakehouserecoverycenter.com/blog/keep-yourself-busy-to-keep-yourself-sober/

SUBSTANCE ABUSE, OPIOIDS

CRISIS, ADDICTION, AND THE WAY OUT

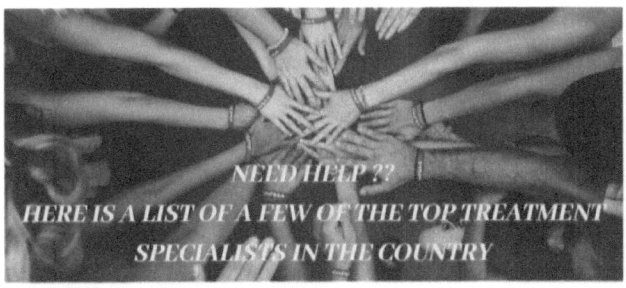

THE LIST INCLUDES:

- *Nationally renowned treatment providers*
- *One-click linked portal access*
- *Locations and contact information*
- *Things to remember when seeking or providing help*

It's one thing to need help, and another to know where to go......

To receive your Renowned Treatment List, visit the link:

<u>Renowned Treatment List</u>

INTRODUCTION

"One of the hardest things was learning that I was worth recovery."

— DEMI LOVATO

The relentless desire for self-gratification is, without a doubt, one of the most striking characteristics of modern society. Since we live in a world that glorifies instant pleasure over hard work and discipline, it is no secret that our society places very little value in the virtues of integrity, self-drive, and personal fulfillment. This obsession with self-indulgence has completely overtaken our innate desire for self-development and personal achievement, thereby leaving us empty and bereft of happiness. Consequently, many people resort to the use of various substances in a bid to get an "instant fix" and feel better about themselves. The result is an engineered drug crisis that has destroyed the lives of many promising individuals who would otherwise be effective assets in our society.

While most people get involved with drugs as a means of escape from the pressures and anxieties of life, they quickly realize that these substances do not provide permanent relief or solutions to the problems that confront them.

Obviously, there is a temporary sense of comfort that these substances provide. This is often a facade, however, that quickly dissipates as soon as the effects of the drug wear off. Nevertheless, during the state of euphoria - which is aroused by the influence of these substances - most people fail to realize the risks and dangers that these drugs present, key of which is addiction.

The problem of substance dependency and addiction is one that has ravaged the lives of millions of people and continues to do so to many more. Medical studies have revealed that at least 40 million Americans aged 12 and older - more than 1 in 7 people - abuse or are addicted to nicotine, alcohol, or other drugs. This number is significantly higher than that of Americans suffering from heart conditions, diabetes, and cancer. Drug addiction is considered a major health crisis not only in America but throughout the world. That is why many governments are adopting increasingly radical measures in a bid to fight this scourge.

Generally, the drugs that have historically been known to contribute to high levels of addiction include marijuana and cocaine. In recent years, however, opioids such as oxycodone have become more central in the global drug crisis. This is mainly attributed to the ease with which these drugs can be acquired.

Furthermore, there is a lack of awareness of the side effects of these substances leading many people to wrongly assume that they are harmless. This misconception couldn't be further from the truth.

According to the US Department of Health and Human Services, more than 130 people died everyday from opioid-related overdoses between the years 2016 and 2017. Reports also showed that opioid-related fatalities accounted for more than half of all drug overdoses in the same year. These statistics undoubtedly paint a very grim picture of the drug crises that have ravaged the world.

If you have fallen victim to substance abuse, you may feel like all hope is lost and that you've sunk too low to pull yourself out of your drug problem. This is not necessarily the case. By making a bold decision and applying the right strategies, you can overcome the problem of opioid addiction and reclaim your health and productivity. Obviously, getting rid of any kind of addiction can be extremely challenging. But with the right state of mind and a genuine resolve, you can completely let go of your addiction problem and come out of the other side a clean, whole, and healthy individual. It is never too late to give up the self-destructive habit of drug use and abuse, and in doing so, improve your overall quality of life in a major way.

Over the course of my long and illustrious career as a self-help author and speaker, I have encountered many individuals who have suffered from opioid addiction and observed the toll it took on their lives. I spent a number of years immersed in extensive research in this area and worked closely with individuals and organizations that have helped broaden my knowledge on opioid addiction. Through scientific study and anecdotal evidence, I have compiled a comprehensive manual on how to completely overcome drug addiction and improve your quality of life. I am very pleased by the positive reviews I have received from people who have applied my method, and in doing so, managed to beat their opioid addiction. I have no doubt whatsoever that the wisdom contained in this book will be a great resource in the battle with drug addiction.

Some of the important lessons that I cover in this book include:

- The specific human experiences that contribute to opioid addiction
- The **two treacherous faces of opioids,** and why you need to be careful

- The 5 things you should always ask your doctor before taking any narcotics
- The **3 risk factors** that very few people are aware of when it comes to opiates
- Reasons that push people to use drugs, and how to get them to stop
- The top **signs of addiction you SHOULDN'T miss** to protect your loved ones
- How to be **quick and alert** in responding to withdrawal symptoms and **avoid a fatal** overdose

While drug addiction is a serious cause for concern, you need not get overly anxious or worried even if you are particularly affected by this scourge. By maintaining the right mindset, you will be able to garner the strength you need to completely beat the opioid problem and start living a healthier life today.

It is also important to note that addiction is an illness like any other, and the people affected by it deserve love and compassion rather than judgment. Adopting this kind of attitude will allow you to see the problem for what it is and consequently learn how to confront it in productive ways that will guarantee success.

1

THE UNAVOIDABLE HUMAN EXPERIENCE

Everyone has experienced pain in one form or another at some point in their lives. It is not too far-fetched to assume that every human being is (to some degree) familiar with the concept of pain. Pain is an integral part not only of our individual perception, but also of our collective human experience.

The science behind pain has been shrouded by mystery despite the universal nature of this condition. Humans throughout history have come up with different theories to explain the existence of pain and the role it plays in our lives. It is only in the past three centuries, however, that scientists and philosophers have developed insights into the nature of pain and devised effective ways of managing it in all its forms.

In this opening chapter, we are going to begin by defining what pain is and embark on an in-depth exploration of its multifaceted nature. Some of the key subjects that we are going to look at include the common perceptions of pain as it manifests in our subjective life experiences as well as the different types of pain human beings encounter. Furthermore, this chapter will provide a brief history of pain management in order to set a background for a study of modern pain relief practices and techniques. Finally, we will look at the correlation between pain and substance abuse which will set the tone for the subsequent chapters of this book.

Commonly Held Conceptions of Pain

Since the dawn of mankind, pain has been a dominant condition and an overarching aspect of the human experience. Ancient civilizations had different conceptions of pain, which guided their understanding of it and the kind of actions they sought to provide relief. Until recently, however, the nature of pain was not well understood. For the purposes of this book, it is important for us to define what pain is and the different ways in which it is perceived.

Pain is fundamentally a primal sensation belonging to a class known as bodily sensations. Other bodily sensations that belong in the same category include tingles, orgasms, and itches. Pain, like all other bodily sensations, is localized in specific parts of one's body at any given time. In addition to this, the sensation of pain is characterized by a distinct intensity and duration relative to certain physical objects (body organs in this case). Another feature of pain that is shared by other bodily sensations is its intimate or subjective nature, meaning that only the individual afflicted by pain is privy to all of its attributes, including its intensity and duration.

This multidimensional nature of pain has led many thinkers and scientists to draw a paradoxical conclusion about pain, namely that it is both a physical object present in the body and simultaneously a metaphysical self-intimating condition that is impossible to quantify. As we are going to see in subsequent chapters of this book, pain straddles both physical and non-physical reality in a very complicated relationship between the body and the mind.

The commonly held conception of pain is one that everyone is familiar with largely because of its epistemic immediacy. In this conception of pain, there are two threads that appear to pull in different directions, thereby giving rise to an act-object duality, which informs our ordinary experience and perception of pain.

In the first thread of commonly held perceptions, pain is regarded as a specific condition of particular body parts or organs. This perception of pain is typically reflected in a localized description of pain. For instance, when one says, "I have an ache in my left shoulder," or, "I feel a sharp pain in my left thumb," one is describing pain as a specific condition of certain localized body parts or organs. In this example, pain is described using straightforward perceptual statements.

This understanding of pain essentially treats the characteristics of pain as if they're the objects of our perceptions. They also prompt us to focus our attention on those specific body locations in a bid to relieve the pain or reduce its intensity. If you have a toothache, for example, you will take the necessary measures to get rid of the pain either through medication or other types of treatment.

While the commonly held conception of pain seems to point to a localized description of pain, it paradoxically stops short of attributing the pain to a physical object or condition. Although one may feel the sensation of pain in a specific part of their body, they do not perceive it as arising from a specific object within the body part. This resistance of attributing pain to a physical object inside the body is informed by the second thread of our commonly held conception of pain, namely, that pain is a subjective experience.

As a subjective experience, pains are considered to be experiences in themselves rather than objects of perceptual experience. This commonly held perception of pain is more dominant and almost universally regarded as the scientific definition of pain. By following this thread of thought, pain can be described as an unpleasant sensation or emotional experience that arises out of intense or damaging stimuli. It is, however, important to note that pain, by its very definition, is subjective in nature and a person's understanding of this phenomenon is shaped by their unique experiences of injury in the early stages of their lives.

The subjective commonly held conception of pain encapsulates both the physical sensation that is brought about by injury as well as the inevitable emotional experience that follows from it. In order for a certain experience to qualify as painful, there has to be an unpleasant sensation as well as an emotional response. In this subjective conception, pain is always considered as a psychological state rather than an actual physical object within a localized body part of an individual. This, as you can see, is in sharp contrast to the first conception, which regards pain as being purely descriptive of a specific physical condition with distinctive spatio-temporal characteristics.

When we describe our experiences of pain, we normally talk about 'feeling' them. The implication is that they are physical objects inside our bodies and we are privy to them through inner perception that is largely due to the private and self-intimating nature of this phenomenon. Furthermore, it points to the intricate way in which our physical bodies are connected to our mental processes. The quality of pain, being a private affair, means that no one can have knowledge of or access to the pain of another individual apart from the individual who is experiencing the pain and expressing it. Even two people who are subjected to the same unpleasant sensation, for instance, two terminally ill cancer patients, will each have unique insights and perceptions of the pain.

Pain is also considered to be subjective because it depends on the perception of an individual for its existence. In other words, pain cannot exist unless it is 'felt' by an individual. Very often, when we express our sympathy to other people for their painful experiences, we tend to say that we "feel their pain." While this is not morally wrong or unethical, it is fundamentally incorrect. Only the individual who is afflicted by the unpleasant sensations that arise from injury or damage and the mental discomfort that comes with it can claim any real authority on their pain. In the same breath, only the people who are directly affected by pain can provide infallible reports about their experience of the same.

The self-intimating nature of pain makes it impossible for there to be a disconnect between the appearance of pain and the reality of it. This means as long as an individual is in the same psychological situation that they would be in if they were in pain, then they are in pain. Conversely, if a person is faced with the same psychological situation that they would have in the absence of pain, then they are not in pain. Since there is no distinction between the appearance of pain and its reality, it is highly unlikely or even impossible for an individual to be mistaken in their judgments of their own pain.

TYPES OF PAIN

Now that we have demystified the commonly held conception of pain, let us look at the main categories of pain that we usually encounter as human beings. Notably, pain can be categorized into three main types: nociceptive pain, neuropathic pain, and psychogenic pain.

Nociceptive Pain

Nociceptive pain is by-and-large the most common type of pain that we experience as human beings. It arises when harmful stimuli are detected by pain receptors known as nociceptors. Nociceptors typically register pain in case a body part is affected by injury or physical damage. This includes injuries such as cuts, bruises, and fractures. Nociceptors are also able to detect thermal and chemical damage.

When there is an injury to a certain part of the body, the nociceptors are stimulated and they promptly send electric signals to the brain through the central nervous system. The brain then processes the information and perceives it as pain; this helps to protect the affected area from further harm or damage.

Nociceptive pain can be classified as chronic or acute, depending on the cause of the pain and its intensity. Most chronic illnesses such as cancer and arthritis often cause recurrent pain which may render a victim incapacitated. Since some of these medical conditions are untreatable, the pain is usually mitigated or suppressed through palliative care with the help of opiates such as morphine.

Nociceptive pain is also commonly classified as either somatic or visceral pain. Somatic pain originates from the nociceptors that are found on the surface of the body and in musculoskeletal tissues. This type of nociceptive pain can be experienced on the skin, tissue, and muscles. Most somatic pains tend to be localized to specific parts of the body and often get worse during physical activities. The pain can, however, be significantly eased through rest.

Visceral pain, on the other hand, arises when the receptors of internal body tissues and organs are activated as a result of injury or damage. Unlike somatic pain which is localized, visceral pain is usually vague, meaning it is difficult to pinpoint any specific part of the body where it arises. This type of pain is often described as a feeling of pressure or ache in the pelvis or abdomen. Some of the events that may trigger visceral pain include distention of hollow organs such as intestines and contraction of visceral muscles. Mild cases of visceral pain can be relieved using over-the-counter painkillers. In cases where significant organ damage has occurred, however, more serious treatments such as surgeries may be required.

Neuropathic Pain

This is a type of pain that is perceptible even when the affected area is exposed to non-painful stimuli. Moreover, it can manifest continuously or in the form of paroxysms. Some of the common features of neuropathic pain in the affected area may include a burning feeling or coldness, itching, and sharp prickly sensations.

The main cause of neuropathic pain is nerve damage that can be caused by an illness such as diabetes, viral infections, and in some cases, surgical procedures. This type of pain is often very difficult to treat and most people only end up achieving some form of partial relief. Nevertheless, there are several treatments that can be recommended to an individual who is experiencing extreme neuropathic pain. These include anticonvulsants such as pregabalin and gabapentin, as well as opioid analgesics.

Psychogenic Pain

Unlike the previous types of pain, psychogenic pain is not an official diagnostic term for pain. The term is, however, commonly used descriptively for pain that is caused or aggravated by mental disturbances such as stress, anxiety, and depression. Some of the common examples of psychogenic pain include headaches, stomach pains, and backaches.

This pain is usually caused by emotional events such as grief, heartbreak, and lovesickness. In some people, it may also be triggered by mental disorders such as bipolar disorder and depression.

Psychogenic pain is often a subject of controversy since there are no physical, sensory damages that are attributed to it. Many people consider it as unreal, thereby stigmatizing the sufferers of this type of pain. Nevertheless, some experts on the subject believe that the purpose of psychogenic pain is to provide a distraction so that extreme emotions which have been suppressed in the subconscious do not surface.

A BRIEF HISTORY OF PAIN MANAGEMENT

Throughout history, humans of all civilizations have sought to find ways to soothe pain or cure it completely. In most ancient societies, pain was generally regarded as a punishment inflicted on humans by the gods for their misdemeanors. To appease the gods and soften their wrath, humans often conducted rituals, which included some kind of animal sacrifice being offered up as atonement. In other cultures, such as the American Indians, various kinds of paraphernalia such as gongs and rattles were used to chase away spirits believed to cause pain inside a person's body.

As primitive forms of medicine began to evolve, healers started using more enhanced, albeit crude forms of treatment to soothe pain. One of the most common techniques that was adopted as a pain-relief mechanism is trepanation. This involved drilling a small hole through a patient's skull to get rid of pain arising from migraines, intracranial diseases, and other serious cranial injuries. While the effectiveness of this procedure in curing pain is largely unknown today, the fact that it was practiced in several cultures, including the Incas and Greeks, suggests that it enjoyed a reasonable degree of success.

Other ancient civilizations pioneered pain-relief techniques and treatments that would later be adopted by modern societies. Ancient Egyptian healers, for instance, were known for fetching electric eels from the Nile and placing them over the wounds of their patients to relieve their pain. A modern version of this pain-relief method (also known as transcutaneous electric nerve stimulation) is used today to treat arthritis pains and backaches.

The use of plant-based remedies to treat pain became popular in Medieval times. A wide variety of herbs was used to cure all sorts of pains, including those arising from underlying health conditions and injuries. In most cases, the herbal medicines contained dozens of different compounds, including opiates.

During the 19th and early 20th centuries, various treatments emerged involving the use of magnets and electricity to treat pain. These treatments were more often than not devised by quacks who were too eager to make some quick money from the gullibility of others. At the same time, there were other commercially available remedies that contained varying amounts of opiates or alcohol. These types of treatment were used particularly to provide temporary relief for pain during medical procedures.

The first significant development in pain relief and treatment came in 1846 when William T.G Morton, a dentist from Boston, and John Collins Warren, a surgeon, performed the first successful surgery with anesthesia. This achievement was an important milestone because it eradicated the pain of surgery, which had been one of mankind's biggest fears. Since then, millions of successful surgical procedures have been performed throughout the world and anesthesia has become a key element of modern surgical practice.

PAIN AND SUBSTANCE ABUSE

Chronic pain can be a very debilitating condition for anyone. It can strain your mobility and hinder your ability to work or exercise. Being in constant pain can also affect your mental state and contribute to illnesses such as depression and anxiety. It is not surprising that many people who are afflicted by chronic pain are at high risk of substance abuse.

Most individuals often turn to drugs as a means of alleviating the pain they are experiencing. For those who are already struggling with substance addiction, the use of medicine to soothe pain can be a very complicated process. Some may turn to alcohol and other drugs such as opiates to find relief for their pain. While drugs and alcohol may provide temporary distractions from pain, they are not very effective in the long run and may even be more damaging to the individual than the actual pain that they are trying to mitigate.

Substance abuse can interfere with one's sleeping patterns and exacerbate mental problems such as anxiety and depression. If the dependency on drugs is not checked, it can wreak havoc on an individual's personal life and mess up their careers. Frequent drug users may also find it difficult to take care of themselves and their families. This can negatively affect their relationships with their loved ones and worsen their situation further.

The treatment of chronic pain, in itself, can also contribute to serious drug dependency issues and addiction. Most doctors often prescribe opiate medications such as Oxycodone and Hydrocodone for pain relief. While the chances of developing an addiction to these drugs is quite low, it is by no means non-existent. Patients who have a history of addiction are particularly at risk of developing a dependency on these drugs. Even those who have no prior history can still become addicted to these drugs due to the fact that they are easily accessible. Moreover, it is easy for patients to exceed the recommended dose due to a desperate need for relieving their chronic pain. This can significantly heighten the risk of developing an addiction to these opioid medications.

The fact that these drugs often induce a 'high' mental state and a calming effect on the body usually prompts patients to seek them out in order to relive that experience. As a result, they become addicted to that feeling and end up dependent on these drugs to function in their ordinary lives.

In light of these concerns, some medical practitioners and primary care physicians have been compelled to find alternative methods of pain management to alleviate their patients' chronic pain. Some of the options that have been suggested include non-drug pain relief methods such as acupuncture, chiropractic treatment, and mind-body therapies. These treatments are highly effective when it comes to the management of chronic pain, and are also considered much safer than opioid medications.

Obviously, there are instances where opiate-based drugs may be more beneficial for chronic pain management. Due to their high risk for addiction, these medicines should only be used when necessary under the advice and supervision of qualified physicians. Patients who have a history of addiction can also use opioid medications for their chronic pain as long as the prescribed treatment takes into account the necessary measures to address their safety and risk of abuse. Otherwise, they risk relapsing back to substance abuse, which can erode any progress that they may have made in their recovery journey.

PAIN CAN BE CONSTRUCTIVE, TOO

Pain is often a very unpleasant experience. Being in constant pain can severely affect our physical, mental, and emotional wellbeing. Pain can hinder us from living our lives to their fullest potential. It is no surprise that our immediate reaction to pain is to find ways of soothing it or eliminating it completely.

Having the mindset of pain as something completely 'negative' can hinder us from understanding the multifaceted nature of pain, and prevent us from deriving any value from our experiences. Despite its negative implications to our physical and emotional wellbeing, pain can actually be beneficial to us in a number of ways.

One of the main benefits of pain is that it enables us to develop empathy for others. For instance, painful experiences such as terminal illness, mental distress, and personal loss can force us to investigate the dynamics of our lives and put into perspective the scope of our human experience. Through these experiences, we come to the realization that despite our minute differences like cultural background, nationality, education, and profession, the existential problems that confront us are the same. Pain teaches us that at the very core of our humanity, we are all the same and that the various things that separate us, such as race, tribe, and religion, are merely illusions. Thanks to the wisdom that we receive through our experiences of pain, we naturally develop a sense of solidarity with our fellow men and women.

Another key benefit of pain is that it motivates us to establish the support structures and defense systems that are essential to our survival. While physical pain is often an indicator of possible tissue damage, it can also be a sign of harmful lifestyle practices. Smoking, for instance, can lead to chest pains due to lung congestion and serious respiratory problems. Likewise, failure to observe a healthy diet and exercise can lead to unhealthy body weight and cause physical pain due to strain on the joints and muscles. While it is always good to take preemptive measures to safeguard our health, sometimes the pain that we experience can be the wake-up call that we need to change our lifestyles and start living better.

Similarly, the emotional and psychological pain that we experience due to unhealthy relationships and loneliness can force us to re-evaluate ourselves and identify the problems that are holding us back. In doing so, we can learn from our mistakes and adopt healthy habits and practises that enable us to build meaningful and satisfying relationships with others. This will help you achieve a greater sense of peace, contentment, and wellbeing.

Another possible benefit of pain is that it helps in character development. Notably, the experience of pain, by virtue of its unpleasantness, pushes us to the limits of our being. This can be a very uncomfortable and distressing thing to go through, that is why most people tend to despair when they are afflicted by pain. Maintaining a positive attitude even when faced with chronic pain and adversity can allow you to develop virtues such as perseverance, patience, and self-discipline. It can also teach us to be more restrained with our desires and appetite, thereby making us mentally stronger and more resilient individuals.

It is important to remember that pain is temporary and transient. No kind of pain, regardless of how chronic it might be, lasts forever. By adopting a positive mindset towards pain, you will be able to muster the strength needed to deal with the discomfort with the hope that one day it shall all pass. Doing so will empower you to persevere through your pain and emerge from the other side as a better person.

In summary, here are some of the main takeaways from this chapter:

- Pain is an indicator of tissue damage and an important bodily sensation that alerts us of physical danger.
- The sensation of pain has a physical component as well as an emotional response.
- Pain is a highly subjective experience; its existence depends on the perception of an individual.
- The experience of pain can be constructive because it allows one to build their character and to develop important virtues such as perseverance, empathy, and patience.

2

ADDICTION AND STIGMA

Whether physical, emotional or psychological, pain can be a very difficult problem to deal with. Normally, when most people experience pain, they look for various ways to try and mitigate it. One of the strategies that they may adopt is the use of prescription opioids to manage or soothe their pain. While the use of opioid drugs may provide temporary relief from pain, this habit often leads to the problems of dependence and addiction, which can take a serious toll on one's health and life.

When we discuss the problem of addiction, we look at how it emerges and progresses, and why it is such a big problem when it comes to effective pain management. More importantly, we will look at the stigma that surrounds and labels addiction and why it is harmful to individuals who are trying to quit taking drugs. We will also cover some of the best strategies of combating addiction stigma in order to create a safe and supportive environment for those trying to quit drugs.

REASONS WHY PEOPLE START TAKING DRUGS

There are numerous factors that make certain people more predisposed to drug-taking. These include:

Genetic Factors

Genetics often plays a role in shaping people's preferences for drugs. Moreover, the interaction between genetics and social factors can make some individuals more predisposed to drug use than others. Children of alcoholic parents, for example, are at a much higher risk of alcohol use and abuse.

Cultural Norms

An individual's preference for drugs is often shaped by the cultural norms and values of the society in which they live. In much of the western world, for instance, the use of drugs and alcohol in universities and colleges is a well-known phenomenon and most campuses lack stringent policies to control their use.

Financial Means

Studies have shown that there is a relationship between financial ability and propensity for drug-taking. For instance, states that have lenient tax laws on drugs usually have higher numbers of drug users. Similarly, states that have higher taxes on drugs such as cigarettes and alcohol tend to have reduced rates of alcoholism and drug-taking.

Self-Medication

Individuals who suffer from chronic pain are often required to take opiate-based prescription drugs to relieve the pain. Even though these drugs are prescribed by a doctor, the resulting addiction and drug dependency cases make it very difficult for those addicted to function without the use of their prescription. Likewise, some people resort to taking alcohol and drugs such as marijuana to cope with emotional and psychological pain.

Personal Temperament

The propensity for drug use is closely related to the personality of an individual. In essence, people who are impulsive by nature tend to value immediate gratification more than delayed rewards, and are likely to take drugs to chase the 'high' feeling without considering the long-term risks involved.

EFFECTS OF DRUG ABUSE ON THE BODY AND BRAIN

Drugs are chemical substances that can have tremendous effects on one's body and psychological state. Most drugs usually have long-lasting health implications, and their effects can be seen long after one has stopped taking them. Although some drugs can have positive health benefits, others can be very damaging to one's mental state. This is especially true if the drugs are used contrary to the recommendation of a physician.

Here are some of the effects of drug abuse:

- Suppressed immunity and increased risk of illness
- Increased risk of heart conditions and possible heart failure
- Lack of appetite due to nausea, which can lead to weight loss
- Lung disease, especially if one has been in taking the drugs by smoking
- Increased chances of having seizures and strokes
- Poor memory and problems with decision-making

The most severe effect of drug abuse on the body is death, which often occurs due to overdose. In the US alone, it is estimated that at least 100 people die every day due to opioid-related overdose.

Apart from their negative implications on physical health, drugs also have tremendous effects on the brain and mental health. Notably, drugs such as marijuana, cocaine, and heroin affect the brain's reward mechanism, which is connected to the limbic system. The use of these drugs usually causes large amounts of dopamine *(a chemical that regulates mood and feelings of pleasure)* to be released in the brain, and this triggers the 'high' feeling.

Although most people don't anticipate the possibility of getting addicted, the feeling that drugs induce often leads people to get hooked on them. That's why many victims of drug abuse often go to great extremes to get a 'quick fix.'

Common drugs such as alcohol and marijuana can have both shortterm and long-term effects on the brain. Alcohol, for example, interferes with the brain's communication pathways, and can cause drastic changes in one's mood. Marijuana, on the other hand, causes short term memory loss.

Similarly, drug and substance abuse can affect an individual, both in the short term and long term. Some of the effects of substance abuse include:

- Increased paranoia and anxiety
- Aggressive impulses
- Visual and auditory hallucinations
- Impaired judgment
- Lack of self-control

Regular intake of drugs can also lead to addiction if it is not controlled early enough. People who become addicted to drugs usually find it difficult to function without taking the substances that they are addicted to. This is why giving up drugs can be a huge challenge for most people. Due to lack of awareness, people tend to demonize drug users and castigate them for taking drugs when, in fact, the drug users are themselves victims of drugs. By understanding how addiction works, and why it is such a huge challenge, we can change our attitude towards victims of substance abuse and become more compassionate towards and supportive of them.

ADDICTION IS A DISEASE

In most societies, drug addiction is perceived to be a moral weakness. As a result, drug addicts are often seen as careless and treated with contempt. The fact of the matter is that drug and substance addiction is a disease rather than a person's moral failing. When people start taking drugs, they usually do so with the belief that they are able to control their usage. As they continue taking them, their brains undergo significant changes, and their bodies gradually build up a tolerance for the drug. When this happens, the individual can no longer achieve their desired feeling from their normal intake of these substances. As a result, they begin taking higher amounts of the drugs to achieve the 'high' they are looking for.

Eventually, the chemical changes that are happening in the brain trigger the impulsive and uncontrollable urge to take drugs, and the individuals become addicted. Once this happens, the person is unable to voluntarily choose not to take drugs even if they are aware of the negative effects that the drug is having on their health and wellbeing.

As you already know, addiction typically occurs when a person's brain chemistry has been altered by habitual drug use. Individuals who manifest chronic addiction often find it very difficult to stop using drugs, and can relapse many times when they try to quit. Abstinence from drugs during this stage can cause serious withdrawal effects, and makes it very hard for addicts to stop taking drugs. In light of this, it is important for drug addiction to be treated as an illness that requires patients to be provided with intensive treatment and support.

People who consider addiction not to be a disease often believe that the problem originates from an individual's life choices. While this might be the case, it is not an entirely truthful or comprehensive assessment. Although a person may have control over their use of drugs *(in the initial stages)*, once they become addicted, they may end up acting in ways that go against their values and beliefs.

Other individuals insist that addiction is not a disease, simply because it can be treated by abstaining from drugs. This could not be further from the truth. For most drug addicts, the effects of abstaining from drugs can be far more serious and dangerous than taking them. In order to rehabilitate themselves from drugs, users are required to go through intensive treatment and lifelong management, similar to people who suffer from chronic conditions such as diabetes and arthritis.

Drug addiction, just like any other illness, usually comes with its own fair share of symptoms. Some of the signs of addiction include:

- Extreme weight loss or gain
- Significant changes in appearance and body hygiene
- Dilated pupils
- Poor psychomotor coordination
- Slurred speech
- Drastic and unexpected changes in mood
- Increased irritability
- Lack of interest and motivation

Due to the lack of understanding about drug and substance abuse, many victims are often stigmatized and treated with contempt. This further exacerbates the use of drugs, since the users may feel isolated and cast-out. In order to help people who are addicted to drugs, a change of mindset is very important. In essence, drug abuse should be treated as an illness that can be cured with the right strategies and support.

FACTORS THAT CONTRIBUTE TO DRUG ADDICTION

Addiction is a very individualistic illness that can be brought about by a number of factors. Some of the main issues that contribute to substance abuse and addiction include:

Trauma

The traumatic events that an individual goes through in their lives often play a role in catalyzing an addiction problem. People who have undergone traumas such as neglect, abuse, and accidents are likely to turn to drugs as a means to ease their pain.

Mental Illness

Studies have shown a strong correlation between mental illness and substance abuse. Most individuals who take drugs usually do so to relieve themselves of stress, anxiety, and feelings of hopelessness that they feel. Conversely, the use of drugs can trigger mental illness or even exacerbate any pre-existing mental problems that one may be suffering from.

Environment

The environment in which one is brought up in can also contribute to substance abuse later in life. Children who are raised by parents who fight a lot, for instance, may resort to drug use to cope with the feelings of anger and neglect that they are experiencing. Similarly, individuals who are brought up by parents who use drugs may be inclined to start taking drugs themselves due to a normalized perception of drugs.

Pressure and Influence from Peers

While peer pressure is usually associated with children and teenagers, adults can also fall victim to the influence of people around them. If one spends time around friends who take drugs, for instance, they can be lured into doing the same as a way of bonding. This can lead to drug abuse and, subsequently, addiction.

FIGHTING ADDICTION STIGMA

Addiction stigma refers to the negative perceptions and beliefs that people hold about drug addicts. Studies have shown that stigma contributes to mental health problems in victims of drug abuse and addiction, and can interfere with their lifestyle. This means any form of discrimination and prejudice can negatively affect their self-esteem, damage their relationships with other people, and even hinder them from accessing treatment. In some cases, the stigma can drive them to commit suicide.

Addiction stigma is often perpetrated by friends and family of the victims of drug abuse. They may judge the person harshly and use dehumanizing terms such as 'junkie' and 'crackhead' to denigrate them. People who do this often wrongly assume that the individual struggling with addiction is irresponsible. They may even be inclined to conclude that the person enjoys being in that condition. This perception could not be further from the truth. Drug addiction, as we have seen, is a serious disease that robs the victim of the ability to make rational choices. Individuals who are struggling with drug addiction need to be accorded support, understanding, and love, instead of judgment and prejudice.

Most individuals who perpetrate stigma against victims of drug addiction often don't realize the damaging effects their habits have on people who are trying to quit drugs. The stigma can have very serious social and emotional implications on individuals affected by addiction. They may feel isolated, marginalized, and lonely, and this can lead to problems such as depression and can increase the potential for self-harm and suicide.

Constant discrimination may also cause victims of drug use to conceal their problems and avoid seeking help. This can further exacerbate the problem and fuel their drug use. When individuals are stigmatized by society due to their drug addiction, they may get stuck in a cycle of drug abuse. In order to help addiction victims overcome their unhealthy habits, it is important to get rid of all stigma that is associated with substance abuse. The question remains: how can we achieve this?

We need to be more open about drug addiction, recovery, and treatment. Granted, talking about addiction can be an uncomfortable experience, especially if a close ally is the victim. Speaking about these difficult problems, however, can help us to personify it and start empathizing with the victims.

We can also end the stigma surrounding addiction by changing the language we use when speaking about it. In our society, drug addiction is often considered as an outcome of poor decision making, and victims are often tagged with demeaning terms such as 'loser' or 'druggie.' This can seriously damage their self worth and confidence, and make them feel hopeless. Instead of chastising drug addicts using these derogatory terms, it is more prudent to address the problem of addiction as a disease that anyone can be afflicted by.

Similarly, we can cast aside stigma by encouraging those who struggle with drug abuse to seek professional treatment. Unfortunately, we live in a world where asking for help is often seen as a weakness. As mentioned before, this can discourage individuals who struggle with addiction from speaking about their situation. By changing our mindset about addiction, however, we can begin to see drug abuse as a serious health problem, thus incentivizing victims to seek treatment.

A lot still remains to be done when it comes to handling addiction stigma. By changing our perception about drug use and abuse, we can let go of the misconceptions we hold and become more inclined towards treatment and recovery.

This chapter has certainly provided valuable insights into the nature of addiction and the stigma around it. As we conclude this segment, here are some of the key takeaways that we would do well to keep in mind:

- Addiction is a disease that requires professional treatment. Victims should be treated with empathy and provided with the support they need on their journey to recovery.
- There are several factors that may contribute to drug abuse and addiction. These include environmental factors, genetic factors, traumas, and mental health issues.
- Stigma from family, friends, and society can be very damaging to the mental wellbeing of individuals who are struggling with drugs, and this stigma can hinder them from seeking treatment.
- Changing our perceptions about drug addiction can help the fight against stigma and motivate victims to seek the help they need to recover. This will help avoid fatalities and extreme cases of opioid addiction.

OPIOIDS AND WHY BE SKEPTICAL

For nearly two decades, the U.S. has been embroiled in a serious opioid crisis that has, to date, claimed hundreds of thousands of lives. The staggering number of deaths related to opioid overdose prompted the Health and Human Services (HHS) to declare a national health emergency and announce various strategies to mitigate the crisis.

Opium, the drug from which opioids are derived, became available in the United States in 1775. During the civil war in the 1860s, the drug was mainly used to treat injured soldiers. As a result, 400,000 soldiers (who had been given morphine) became addicted. By the late 1800s, the rate of opioid addiction had increased significantly due to the over-the-counter availability of opioids. In the early 1900s, morphine became the most commonly prescribed drug for pain management. At the same time, many people started using opioid drugs recreationally, by crushing the pills and inhaling them.

In order to limit the recreational use of opioid drugs, the Harrison Narcotics Act made opioids available only by prescription. In the years beginning 1920 to 1950, opioids were exclusively prescribed to patients who were dying for their acute pain rather than chronic pain.

This was done in order to avoid addiction. By the early 1970s, there was a lot of stigma and fear associated with opioid addiction. As a result, doctors started to opt for surgery and other non-pharmaceutical treatment for chronic pain.

From 1970 to 1990, the American Pain Society advocated for the use of non-addictive therapies to treat cancer-related pain. The FDA also approved the use of Vicodin and Percocet for the decade starting 1976 to 1986. In 1986, however, the World Health Organization (WHO) created a set of guidelines to treat cancer patients. The organization recommended that opioids be used to treat chronic pain in cancer patients only if no other treatment options were available. Between the years 1997 to 2002, there was a sharp rise in the number of prescriptions for opioid drugs. Morphine prescriptions increased by 73% and hydromorphone by 96% whereas the prescriptions for fentanyl and Oxycodone spiked by 226% and 402% respectively.

By the mid-2000s, there were numerous reports of teenagers starting to use opioids obtained from their parent's prescriptions. Heroin also became available and started being used illicitly. In 2013, there were an estimated 23 000 drug-dependent babies who were born with Neonatal Abstinence Syndrome. Two years later, the number of reported opioid overdose deaths had increased to 52 404. Currently, the death rate from opioid overdose is 142 every single day.

The trajectory of opioid-related deaths can be documented in three phases. The first phase began in the early 1990s when pharmaceutical companies declared that patients would not become addicted to opioid prescription drugs. This provided an incentive for health providers to prescribe these drugs to patients. As a result, the number of opioid overdoses started increasing dramatically in the late 1990s.

The second phase of the opioid crisis started in 2010 when the use of heroin skyrocketed in the U.S. This led to a rapid increase in overdose-related deaths, which claimed thousands. In 2013, the opioid crisis entered its third phase with a significant increase in the number of opioid-related deaths involving illegal synthetic opioids such as fentanyl. The market for fentanyl has been steadily growing ever since despite government efforts to clamp down on the illegal drug trade.

The perpetuation of the opioid crisis has been mainly facilitated by a lack of information and awareness about these drugs and the dangers they pose. Pharmaceutical companies, for instance, have been complicit in this health crisis by downplaying the harmful effects of the drugs, and encouraging health providers to continue prescribing them.

Let us now explore the topic of opioids, what they are, and why they are very central to the health disaster that we've been facing for more than two decades.

What are Opioids?

Opioids are a class of drugs that are derived from the opium poppy plant. While most opioids are used as prescription drugs, some types of opioids are purely used for recreational purposes.

Opioids work by inhibiting the pain signals between the body and the brain. That's why they are usually administered as painkillers to patients who are suffering from chronic pain. These drugs can also induce a relaxing and calming 'high' feeling, which makes them highly addictive.

Opioids are commonly referred to as narcotics. This is because they don't belong in the same class as other painkillers like Tylenol and aspirin, even though they do have the same pain relief properties. Although these drugs are often prescribed for use by medical practitioners, they are not entirely safe. As a matter of fact, opioids tend to have very serious side effects.

Some of the short-term health effects of opioids include:

- Drowsiness

- Mental fog
- Constipation
- Shallow breathing
- Nausea
- Unconsciousness

Frequent use of prescription opioids can lead to increased tolerance and dependence. As a result, patients may find that they require higher quantities each time in order to achieve the desired effect. This can eventually lead to addiction, which is clinically referred to as 'opioid use disorder.'

When taken at very high doses, opioids can lead to breathing complications or even death. It is worth noting that the risk of respiratory distress is much higher for people who are taking opioids for the first time, and those that are using medications that are known to react with these drugs.

Due to the severity of the risks involved, opioids should only be used for pain relief in cases where no other type of treatment is available. In addition to this, you should only use opioids as directed by a qualified physician, and you need to inform them about any pre-existing medical conditions that you may have, as well as any other drugs you may be using.

Types of Opioids

While the term 'opioid' is generally used to describe different types of drugs that are derived from the opium poppy plant, drugs that fall under this category have various differences. As such, they are further grouped depending on how they are made or acquired. Under this classification criterion, there are three categories of opioids, namely: Semi-synthetic opioids, fully synthetic opioids, and natural opiates.

Semi-synthetic opioids are a class of drugs that are manufactured artificially in medical labs using opiate compounds. Some of the well-known examples of these man-made opioids include drugs such as hydrocodone, oxycodone, and hydromorphone.

Unlike semi-synthetic opioids, which are made using opiate compounds, fully synthetic opioids are manufactured using other chemicals. Some of the drugs that fall in this category include fentanyl, tramadol, methadone, and pethidine.

Natural opiates are alkaloid compounds that occur naturally in the poppy plant. Some of the most common natural opiates include narcotine, codeine, morphine, papaverine, thebaine, and narceine.

Most naturally occurring and semi-synthetic opioids are legal and can be easily acquired from a pharmacy on the recommendations of a medical practitioner. These opioids are usually manufactured by pharmaceutical companies, which are strictly regulated by the government through certain safety standards. Synthetic opioids, on the other hand, are illegally made and sold by black market operators both locally and in foreign countries.

Since the manufacture and sale of synthetic opioid drugs are unregulated, many organizations and individuals who make them often mix harmful chemicals and drugs such as cocaine, methamphetamine, heroin, and MDMA. As a result, synthetic opioids are often far more dangerous and addictive than naturally occurring and semi-synthetic opioids. In fact, the past decade has seen a sharp rise in opioid-related fatalities, which are linked to illegal synthetic drugs such as fentanyl and methadone.

Nevertheless, the fact that prescription opioids such as oxycodone and hydrocodone are manufactured by licensed pharmaceutical companies does not necessarily mean that they are safe. These drugs have also contributed significantly to the opioid crisis and lead to many fatalities as a result of overdose. Some medical experts and observers even argue that these drugs are far more dangerous, owing to the fact that they are legal and easily accessible.

Given the tremendous risks that all the different types of opioids present to users, it is absolutely vital to be adequately informed on the dangers and side effects that these drugs may pose. Having the right information easily accessible can go a long way towards empowering individuals who are at high risk of addiction to make the right decisions when it comes to both legal and illegal opioids.

EFFECTS OF OPIOIDS ON THE BODY

As we have seen from the previous topic, opioids can be classified depending on how they are made. Using this criterion, we can categorize opioid drugs as naturally-occurring, semi-synthetic and fully synthetic. Depending on the manner in which they are derived and manufactured, different types of opioids will have different pharmacological effects.

In this section, we are going to look at the various effects that specific types of opioids have on the body. First, let us briefly go over some of the general effects that opioids tend to produce when ingested or administered:

Analgesic Effects

Opioids are mostly given to patients who are suffering from chronic pain because of the drug's strong analgesic effects. These drugs are highly effective at relieving poorly localized, dull pain that is emanating from deeper body structures such as muscles and organ tissues. Since neuropathic pain may be very persistent, patients often report that opioid medications help them manage it properly until it is almost unnoticeable in some cases. While opioids are quite effective at relieving neuropathic pain, however, they are ineffective when it comes to sharp nociceptive pain from injuries such as cuts on the skin.

Sedative Properties

Opioids are known to induce drowsiness and a relaxed feeling of tranquility. In some instances, the pain-relief properties of opioids are accompanied by sleep, although this is not always the case.

Euphoric and Dysphoric Feelings

Some opiates such as morphine and codeine often induce a feeling of euphoria and contentment when used. This feeling, accompanied by the pain-relief properties of the drugs, usually contributes to the addictive nature of these opioids. On the other hand, some opioids are known to elicit feelings of dysphoria. Even morphine, which is very effective as a pain-reliever, can cause restlessness and agitation in some patients when they realize they are no longer in pain.

Opioid Tolerance and Dependence

Although this phenomenon is not fully understood, many experts believe that increased tolerance to opioids may be as a result of a decrease in the production of endogenous opioids. These are the opioid compounds that are naturally released in the brain.

Another possible explanation for opioid tolerance is the downregulation of opioid receptors, which are responsible for mediating the body's response to different hormones and neurotransmitters.

Apart from increased tolerance, the habitual use of opioids can also lead to dependence - a condition whereby an individual experiences adverse physical symptoms whenever they withdraw from drug usage. Common symptoms that long-term opioid users may manifest include sweating, diarrhea, muscle cramps, vomiting, restlessness, and irritability.

Once a person develops a physical dependence, they may be unable to make rational choices about their drug use even when they are well aware of the implications on their health and wellbeing. This is why opioid dependence and addiction should be viewed and treated as the illness it is.

Rigidity of Muscles

When taken in very large doses, opioids may cause muscles to become more rigid and tense, especially around the thoracic cavity.

Suppressed Immunity

Prolonged opioid use puts the body under a lot of strain, and may lead to suppression of the body's immune system. This puts long-term users at great risk of contracting serious illnesses.

Although different opioids tend to produce similar effects, they differ substantially in a number of ways, most notably, their duration of action. In order to truly appreciate how these drugs work, let us now look at the ways in which some of the most common opioids work.

Morphine

Morphine is a naturally occurring opioid medication that is derived from phenanthrene. It is perhaps the most well-known medicative opioid and is often considered the standard against which all other opioid drugs are measured.

Due to its effectiveness as a pain reliever, morphine is usually prescribed to persons that are suffering from chronic neuropathic pain. The drug can be administered in various ways including orally, intravenously, epidurally, and intramuscularly. Morphine typically has a quick onset of action, which peaks about 60 minutes after the injection has been administered. The drug also has a duration of action of 3-4 hours.

Some of the effects of morphine:

- Strong pain-relief and analgesic properties; that's why it is widely considered as the gold standard of opioid therapy.
- May induce euphoria, dysphoria, and hallucinations.
- Often causes respiratory depression by slowing down breathing.

- May induce nausea and vomiting.

Codeine

Codeine is a naturally occurring opiate and is often administered as a pain-relief medication. Although the actual mechanism of codeine is not fully understood, experts believe that it works by binding to the opioid receptors in the brain. These receptors are responsible for transmitting the sensation of pain in the brain and body. Codeine, however, has a very low affinity for opioid receptors compared to other opioids like morphine and hydrocodone. Patients who take codeine often develop a high tolerance for their pain, although the sensation may still be apparent to them.

In addition to alleviating pain, codeine induces sedation and depresses breathing. The drug is also often combined with other drugs like aspirin and Tylenol to provide more effective pain relief.

Some of the side effects of codeine include:

- Euphoria
- Respiratory depression
- Dizziness
- Vomiting
- Constipation
- Abdominal pain
- Itching
- Rash
- Low blood pressure

Codeine, like all opioids, is an addictive drug. When used for pain relief over short periods of time, a dependency is unlikely although not entirely impossible. People who use the drug over prolonged periods may experience severe effects if the drug is suddenly withdrawn. This is why the dose of codeine should be reduced gradually, instead of sudden withdrawal.

Heroin

Heroin is an illegal opioid drug that is made from morphine, a naturally occurring substance found in the seedpods of certain varieties of the poppy plant. The drug is usually sold as a white or brownish powder or a black substance known as black tar heroin. This semi-synthetic drug is believed to be at least twice as potent as morphine, which makes it highly effective for pain management.

Heroin is usually administered or ingested in several different ways, including sniffing, snorting, and smoking. Once the drug reaches the brain, it is quickly converted into morphine, and rapidly binds to the opioid receptors.

Some of the immediate (short-term) side effects include:

- Drowsiness
- Sedation
- Nausea
- Vomiting
- Respiratory depression
- Slowed heart function

Studies have also shown that habitual heroin usage can affect a patient's brain and their ability to control their actions and make proper judgments.

Fentanyl

Fentanyl is a potent synthetic opioid, which is 50 to 100 times more potent than morphine. It is generally used as an analgesic to relieve chronic pain, especially from surgeries. The drug is also administered to patients experiencing chronic pain due to terminal illness.

Although fentanyl is treated as a prescription opioid, many illegal labs are known to manufacture the drug in the black market and sell it to users who have no doctor's prescription. Some of the street names of fentanyl include China White, Apache, China Girl, Dance Fever, and Murder 8.

The illegal manufacture and sale of fentanyl has been central to the opioid crisis over the past decade. Statistics have shown that more than half of opioid-related fatalities are a result of a fentanyl overdose. People who ingest fentanyl in large doses are likely to experience hypoxia, a condition that reduces the amount of oxygen that reaches the brain. When this happens, users of the drug may suffer permanent brain damage or slip into a coma.

Some of the side effects of fentanyl include:

- Constipation
- Nausea
- Confusion
- Drowsiness
- Breathing problems
- Unconsciousness

Fentanyl overdoses are usually treated using a drug known as Naloxone. This drug acts by binding to the opioid receptors in the brain and inhibiting the action of opiates. Naloxone should be administered immediately after an overdose to inhibit fentanyl action and prevent serious brain damage and fatality. Since fentanyl is many times more potent than morphine or codeine, multiple doses of Naloxone are required to successfully treat fentanyl overdose.

Individuals who are given Naloxone should be closely monitored to ensure their breathing doesn't slow down or stop. The drug is typically administered as an injection or nasal spray.

Since fentanyl is a very addictive opioid, individuals who are hooked on the drug may find it difficult to stop using it. Moreover, sudden withdrawal of the drug may cause serious side effects such as:

- Diarrhea and vomiting
- Lack of sleep
- Uncontrollable body movements
- Severe cravings for fentanyl
- Muscle pain

Treatment for fentanyl usually involves medication and behavioral therapy. Some of the medicines that have been approved for treating fentanyl addiction include methadone and buprenorphine; both function by binding to the opioid receptors in the brain. This helps to reduce the patients' craving for fentanyl. Naltrexone, another commonly used drug, blocks opioid receptors in the brain, thus preventing fentanyl from binding to the brain's receptors.

In addition to medication, counseling is also very crucial in the treatment of fentanyl addiction, to help victims develop positive attitudes and practises in relation to their drug use.

Hydrocodone

Hydrocodone is a prescription opioid that is used to treat all types of pain. Unlike natural opiates like morphine and codeine, which occur naturally, hydrocodone is usually made in a lab. It is often administered to people who have serious injuries, or those that have undergone major procedures. Nevertheless, just like other opioids, hydrocodone is very addictive, and long-term use of the drug can lead to tolerance and dependence.

Some of the most commonly reported side effects of taking hydrocodone include:

- Reduced breathing rate

- Expanded pupils
- Sleepiness
- Slurred speech
- Vomiting
- Nausea
- Constipation
- Confusion
- Itchy skin
- Euphoria

Long-term use of hydrocodone can lead to lasting effects on the brain. Individuals who have developed an addiction for this drug may experience significant mood and behavioral changes. They are also likely to suffer from other health problems such as liver and kidney disease, respiratory stress, insomnia, anxiety, and depression.

Taking large amounts of hydrocodone can easily lead to an overdose. When this happens, the breathing rate of a user can plummet, thereby causing hypoxia (lack of enough oxygen reaching the brain). In severe cases of hydrocodone overdose, fatalities are likely to occur unless the patient receives immediate treatment.

Due to the serious health risks involved, hydrocodone should only be taken under the prescription of a medical professional.

Methadone

Methadone is often prescribed as a pain-relief medication, particularly to patients who have tolerance or adverse reactions to other opiates like morphine and codeine. More commonly, the drug is used to prevent withdrawal effects in patients who are going through treatment for opioid addiction.

It comes in various forms, including dispersible tablets, non-dispersible tablets, and concentrated solutions, and can either be administered orally or intravenously.

Some of the common side effects of methadone include:

- Drowsiness
- Slowed breathing
- Constipation
- Nausea
- Vomiting
- Headaches
- Abdominal Pain
- Dizziness

Although most mild side effects usually dissipate after a few days, the drug may cause more severe effects in some cases including respiratory failure and low blood pressure.

Some of the most common withdrawal effects that users of methadone are likely to experience include:

- Anxiety and irritability
- Restlessness
- Insomnia
- High blood pressure
- Increased breathing rate
- Fast heart rate
- Stomach cramps and diarrhea
- Muscle and back pains

Oxycodone

Oxycodone is a synthetic opioid drug that is commonly administered as a painkiller. It is also one of the most commonly abused prescription drugs in the U.S. Most people who abuse Oxycodone usually start out taking the prescribed dose. Then, as their tolerance with habitual use grows, they start requiring higher doses in order to experience the same effects.

The transition from prescriptive use to addiction can be very quick when it comes to Oxycodone. This is due to the high potency of the drug. Patients who are using it to manage pain due to chronic illnesses may find it difficult to control their use of the drug and end up becoming dependent. Some of the common signs and symptoms of Oxycodone dependence and addiction include:

- Requiring higher doses of the drug to achieve a high
- Experiencing unpleasant symptoms when Oxycodone is withdrawn
- Having intense cravings for the drug when not under the influence of it
- Prioritizing the drug more than anything else in their lives
- Being reckless and not caring about one's safety when using the drug
- Struggling financially since a lot of money is spent on purchasing the drug
- Neglecting relationships with others such as family members and friends

People who are struggling with Oxycodone dependence and addiction usually need to undergo a medical detoxification and continual treatment in order to get off the drug and prevent relapse.

Prolonged use of this drug, especially if not used as recommended by a medical doctor is considered as drug abuse. Individuals who take high doses of the drug either medically or recreationally may experience a wide array of effects, most of which are unpleasant. These include:

- Drowsiness
- Dizziness
- Euphoria
- Hallucinations
- Nausea

- Vomiting
- Reduced anxiety
- Calmness
- Relaxation
- Slowed breathing

Since the use of prescription opioids like Oxycodone is generally accepted in society, identifying and mitigating abuse and addiction can be quite challenging. In cases where users have prescriptions for the drug, it can be difficult to tell the difference between proper use and abuse. It generally boils down to the negative implications that the drug has on the life of the user. Nevertheless, one of the telltale signs of Oxycodone addiction is when a user's prescription typically runs out faster than the expected time. This can imply that the person is using more than the recommended dose of the drug.

It is worth noting that the use of Oxycodone can pose serious health risks to the individual. Like other opioids, Oxycodone usually causes depressed breathing, which may lead to severe medical issues such as unconsciousness, brain damage, and fatality. Even if you are using the drug prescriptively for pain relief, there are a number of safety precautions that you ought to follow. These include:

- Inform your doctor of any allergic reactions you may have to Oxycodone or any other ingredients in the medication you plan to take
- Make sure your doctor or pharmacist is aware of any other medications, vitamins or herbs that you are taking or planning to take concurrently with the Oxycodone medication
- Tell your doctor if you're breastfeeding
- Inform your doctor of any surgical procedures you may have undergone recently

- Do not use any heavy machinery or drive when taking this medication until you know how exactly the drug affects you
- Talk to your doctor about modifying your diet when taking Oxycodone in order to prevent constipation

Patients who are taking Oxycodone are often advised to have the drug Naloxone readily available. This drug is used to block the effects of opioids and reverse their symptoms. In the case of an opioid overdose, Naloxone is usually administered to patients in order to avert damage to the patient's organs and prevent fatality. Since you may not be able to treat yourself in the event of an overdose, you should ensure that your family members, caregivers or roommates know how to identify symptoms of an overdose and how to administer Naloxone in case of an overdose, before emergency services arrive.

Hydromorphone

Hydromorphone is an opioid derivative of morphine which is commonly given as a painkiller medication due to its analgesic properties. This drug is known to bind to different types of brain receptors including mu-opioid, kappa, and delta receptors. Hydromorphone is available in the form of oral tablets sold under brand names such as Exalgo which is an extended-release form and Dilaudid which is an immediate-release version. The onset of release of the immediate release version of hydromorphone is usually achieved in 15 to 20 minutes whereas the extended-release form of the drug may take up to 6 hours to become effective.

Apart from the oral pill forms of the drug, hydromorphone is also available in the form of an injectable solution and an oral liquid solution. This drug is usually prescribed for pain relief purposes in cases where other medications are ineffective. Hydromorphone is also sometimes used together with other medications in combined therapies.

Hydromorphone, like most opioid drugs, induces a wide variety of side effects. Some of the most common symptoms that may be experienced shortly after taking the drug include:

- Drowsiness
- Dizziness
- Insomnia
- Lightheadedness
- Sweating
- Euphoria
- Itching

These mild effects usually taper off or completely disappear after a few days or weeks. In some cases, more severe side effects can be experienced by patients who medicate using hydromorphone. Some of the more adverse side effects of this opioid drug include:

- Increased or slowed down heart rate
- Chest pains
- Vision problems such as blurry vision, double vision, and constricted pupils
- Abdominal discomfort
- Diarrhea
- Involuntary muscle movement
- Drastic changes in mood
- Psychological problems such as anxiety and depression
- Insomnia
- Breathing problems

In order to minimize the risk of adverse symptoms, hydromorphone is to be used in the right amounts.

HOW DO OPIOIDS WORK IN THE BRAIN?

One of the biggest misconceptions about opioid addiction is that individuals abuse these drugs simply to feel the euphoric effects that they are known to induce. Although this perception is not baseless, it does not fully capture the dynamics of opioid action in the brain that leads to addiction. While many individuals start taking opioids to manage pain, the drastic changes that occur in the brain as a result often lead to tolerance and dependency.

How *do* opioid drugs affect the brain?

Generally, opioids act on the brain by binding to the receptors that are responsible for how we perceive sensations such as pleasure and pain. Once an opioid drug such as heroin or codeine is ingested, the enzymes in the brain quickly convert it to morphine, which has pain-relieving properties. The process of binding usually causes large amounts of the hormone dopamine to be released, which is why users often feel euphoric upon taking prescription opioids. The problem with this is that the flood of dopamine in the brain may exceed what the body is normally capable of producing.

As an individual continues to take opioid drugs habitually, the brain begins to adapt to the increased levels of dopamine. Consequently, the body starts to develop a tolerance for the drug. When this happens, frequent opioid users find themselves in need of more drugs to feel normal. At this stage, they have become dependent and addicted to the drug, and their drug use is no longer a conscious decision.

Addiction is undoubtedly one of the serious effects of habitual opioid use on the brain, and can lead to serious mental health problems. Once addiction has taken hold, it can be very difficult for an individual to stop taking opioids due to withdrawal effects. This can significantly increase their drug use and put the victims in a vicious cycle, which could end in serious damage to one's health or even death.

Some of the habits and mental changes that may be brought about by long-term opioid use include:

- Poor memory/forgetfulness
- Inability to regulate one's actions
- Reduced flexibility when it comes to accomplishing tasks
- Diminished reasoning ability
- Poor decision-making skills
- Inability to plan

In most cases, the negative effects of prolonged opioid use are very difficult to reverse. These can take a serious toll on one's overall health and wellbeing, and can increase the risk of developing psychological problems such as anxiety and depression. Once an individual has developed an opioid addiction, it can be very difficult, albeit possible, for them to recover.

Patients who are suffering from addiction often require a multilayered treatment plan, which involves medication as well as counseling. They also need support, not only from their loved ones, but from society at large. With the right help and treatment, recovery from opioid addiction is very possible regardless of the duration of time one has been ailing for.

In conclusion, this chapter has been invaluable in providing an indepth analysis of opioid drugs, how they are made, and the implications that they have on one's mental health. Some of the key takeaways from this chapter include the following:

- There are three main types of opioids, namely, naturally-occurring opiates, semi-synthetic opioids, and fully synthetic opioids
- All opioids work by binding to the brain's receptors, causing dopamine to be produced in very high amounts
- Opioids tend to induce various short term effects, which may

include nausea, vomiting, abdominal pain and discomfort, respiratory distress and many more
- Prolonged use of opioids leads to increased tolerance and dependence, which consequently cause users to become addicted to these drugs
- Opioids use may affect a person's mood, speech and poor memory
- Opioids must be strictly used under the guidance of a qualified medical practitioner to lower the risk of overdose, which may cause serious brain damage or fatality

Given the high risks that opioids expose users to, it is absolutely important for dependency and addiction to be diagnosed early. This can significantly improve the chances of successful treatment, and may lower the risk of serious damage and death.

In the next chapter, we are going to look at some of the tell-tale signs of addiction, and how one can pick on them early before the problem spirals out of control. By doing so, an individual who is suffering from opioid addiction can be provided with the necessary assistance and rehabilitation to fully recover from these drugs.

4

SIGNS OF ADDICTION AND HOW TO NOTICE THEM EARLY

Opioids, like other drugs and medications, are essentially chemical in nature. This means they have the ability to alter our brain and body chemistry in fundamental ways. Notably, they not only have the power to alter how we feel, but also the way we think. It is inevitable, then, that an individual who is dependent on or addicted to these drugs will manifest certain signs and symptoms. Early diagnosis of these symptoms is absolutely important as it makes it possible for treatment to be administered before the condition gets out of hand.

Despite knowing the importance of early detection and treatment, the signs of opioid addiction aren't always very obvious. In cases where individuals are using prescription drugs to manage various kinds of pain, it can be difficult to tell whether the patients are addicted to the drugs or using them pragmatically to soothe their pain. In this chapter, we will cover some of the tell-tale signs of addiction, and how to pick up on them easily. We shall also look at factors that may predispose an individual to opioid addiction.

ADDICTION MODELS

Opioid tolerance, dependence, and addiction are all directly linked to the changes that the brain undergoes when introduced to opioid drugs. When an addict is trying to recover, they are fighting to reverse these changes.

In the early stages of opioid abuse, the stimulatory effects of these drugs on the mesolimbic reward system is what drives individuals to consume them. Once the inclination to use opioids continues to build up, however, users of these drugs may become dependent on them.

In general, the exposure of the brain to opioids interferes with the ability of the body to function optimally on its own. This exposure and interference continues its prompts to take the drugs to achieve the desired effects.

Over the years, various models have been proposed to describe the problem of addiction. Let us now briefly discuss some of these theories, and how they have influenced the understanding and treatment of drug addiction.

Automatic Processing Theories

These models of drug addiction are built around the assumption that addiction is shaped without the need for conscious intentions or decision making. In other words, Automatic Processing Theories explore ideas of addiction happening in the absence of our self-regulatory mechanisms. There are various theories that fall under the Automatic Processing model of drug addiction. They include:

- Learning Theories - These models hold that addiction stems from learning the relationships between responses, cues, and powerful reinforcers, which may be either positive or negative.
- Drive Theories - These link addiction to homeostatic

processes such as cravings, which act as powerful motivating factors for drug use.
- Inhibition Dysfunction Theories - These models propose that addiction is the result of the impairment of regulatory mechanisms, which are meant to control our impulses with regard to drug use.
- Imitation Theories - These models link addiction to the inclination of individuals to imitate the actions of group members.

In response to these models of addiction, treatment is usually predicated on learning alternative practices, avoiding triggering stimuli for drug use, and increasing control of addictive habits. Under these models, treatment is more focused on developing new associations through training and repetition to overcome the problem of drug use. Medication may also be used to block actions that reinforce drug use and stimulate the process of change.

Reflective Choice Theories

These models are based on the assumption that human activities are, to some extent, influenced by a self-conscious evaluation of options and available alternatives. The main Reflective Choice Theories that are used to describe drug addiction are:

- Rational Choice Theory - This model holds that drug addiction is the result of rational choices made by an individual who believes that the benefits of using these addictive drugs far outweigh the cost of doing so.
- Biased Choice Theory - This model of addiction is based on the assumption that whereas an individual does make a reflective choice, they are subject to the effects of factors such as emotions, which may reduce the quality of choice made and even result in counterproductive decisions.

According to this perspective of drug addiction, treatment can be achieved by changing the benefit/cost ratio. This is done by increasing the cost of addictive habits and/or increasing the benefits of non-addictive actions to alter the individual's perception of this ratio.

Goal-Focused Theories

These models place greater emphasis on the goal of addictive practises. Some of the theories that support these models of drug addiction include:

- Positive Reward Theories - The model of Positive Rewards considers the pleasure and satisfaction that arises from drug use as the motivating factor for addiction. These rewards may be induced psychologically; for example, the euphoria that drug users experience when they take these substances. The rewards can also be more objective-based; for instance, taking drugs to alleviate chronic pain.
- Acquired Need Theories - In these models of addiction, the physiological rewards of taking addictive substances are thought to result in habituation and adaptation. The withdrawal effects that result from the habitual use of drugs, and the strong aversion to those effects, is consequently seen as the driving force behind addiction.
- Identity and Identification Theories - These theories on addiction posit that addictive habits may be influenced by the presence of self-destructive or anti-social elements. So, a person who's intent on losing weight, for instance, may be driven to take up smoking as a means of achieving that objective.

From the standpoint of these Goal-Focused Theories, the problem of addiction stems from the desire of an individual to meet certain needs. Successful treatment aims at reducing the pleasure of addictive practices by enhancing one's internal control mechanism via medication.

Another strategy involves counseling designed to help the user to find alternative sources of pleasure and personal fulfillment.

Integrative Theories

Integrative models of drug addiction are built on the premise that drug addiction stems from a complex interrelation of numerous factors, including the environment and the internal state of an individual. These factors interact with automatic or conscious processes targeting pleasure and avoiding physical or mental discomfort. The most common Integrative Theory on drug addiction is the Self-Regulation model. This theory is predicated on the ability of an individual to counteract their immediate reaction towards their desires and impulses. It assumes that a person's ability to counter these impulses may be limited by lack of skills, strategy, and capacity.

Other integrative theories approach the problem of addiction from an even wider scope. These models relate one's habits and traits with the environment and social context in which they exist. Consequently, they try to overcome the limitations of more specific models by integrating the various factors that influence drug addiction in a single unified model.

In light of the broad scope of Integrative models of addiction, treatments tend to make reference to some of the strategies that are commonly employed in more specific models. In this sense, Integrative Theories of substance addiction are generally more inclusive in their approach to treatment options

Biological Theories

In Biological models, addiction is considered to be a disease of the brain under the general assumption that the neural functioning of addicts is very different from that of non-addicts. Biological Theories also hold that various parameters influence the process of drug dependence and addiction including genetics, environmental factors, and physiological factors. Since human behavior is related to brain activity, all these factors are believed to give rise to addiction by acting on the neural processes of an individual's brain.

Under these models, treatment for addiction is focused on medications and therapies that are designed to change the way the brain of an addicted individual operates.

Process of Change Theories

While most models of addiction aim to describe how and why substance addiction develops, the Process of Change Theories mainly focus on how individuals recover. These models endeavor to optimize intervention strategies according to a general step-by-step model of change in an individual's habits and attitudes towards addictive substances. These interventions are usually adapted to the different stages of addiction in order to achieve maximum effect and avoid a relapse.

KNOWN RISK FACTORS OF OPIOID MISUSE AND ADDICTION

Opioid addiction usually happens when these prescription drugs are taken contrary to the recommendations of a physician; for instance, crushing a pill so that it can be snorted. This habit can be very dangerous and life-threatening especially if the drug has a lengthy action period. When the drug is rapidly delivered into the body, an overdose may occur. This can lead to serious damage to organs such as the brain, heart, liver, and may result in fatalities.

Studies have shown that the duration of time in which a person uses prescription opioids may raise the risk of addiction. Using these drugs for more than a few days, for instance, increases the likelihood of habitual use and addiction. There are various other factors that may significantly increase the risk of opioid addiction. These include:

Poverty and Unemployment

The relationship between poverty and drug addiction has been a subject of interest for many years. It is obviously very strange to think that individuals who have a low-income can afford the expensive lifestyle that comes with habitual drug use. Studies have shown, however, that poverty may contribute to drug addiction in a number of ways.

First, people of low socio-economic status are far more likely to abuse drugs than those who are wealthier. This is because when an economy is not thriving, individuals who have no job (and have more time on their hands) are more likely to use drugs. They are consequently at higher risk of becoming addicted than those who have full-time jobs.

Moreover, people who are addicted to drugs and live in poor conditions are less likely to be able to access treatment and rehabilitation centers. This means they are at risk of being hooked on drugs for longer.

Users living in poverty are also likely to get addicted to drugs, since they are more exposed to the drug trade, and may find the sale of drugs to be a lucrative activity. This may make it difficult for them to stay sober.

Family History of Substance Abuse

Studies have shown a correlation between family history and substance addiction. For instance, children who are raised by parents who habitually take drugs are at higher risk of addiction later in life. This is because they are likely to mimic the actions of their caregivers.

Personal History of Substance Abuse

Having a personal history of substance abuse can increase the risk of an individual becoming addicted to opioids. A person who has used drugs in the past may find it much easier to access them. This makes them more likely to become addicted to prescription opioids. Furthermore, individuals who are trying to quit opioids may easily relapse when not provided with the right treatment and support.

Age

Studies have shown that drug abuse and addiction are not limited to a particular age group. Younger individuals may be more inclined to take drugs recreationally due to peer pressure. On the other hand, studies have shown that older individuals (age 65+) who use opioid medications are at greater risk of dying from opioid overdose.

History of Criminal Activity or Legal Problems, Including DUIs

Criminal actions are closely associated with drug addiction. This is due to the fact that when most individuals commit crimes, they are usually under the influence of some kind of drug. For this reason, people who have a history of criminal activities are at greater risk of developing an addiction.

Regular Contact With High-Risk People or High-Risk Environments

Drug addiction is a prevalent problem in low-income neighborhoods where unemployment is rampant, and individuals often have to resort to selling drugs in order to survive. Those who are regularly exposed to high-risk persons such as drug dealers and users are at high risk of becoming addicts themselves.

Mental Disorders

Opioid addiction disorders are often associated with mental disorders. This is because people who suffer from mental illnesses like anxiety and depression are likely to use drugs in a bid to get rid of their pain. Conversely, symptoms of drug addiction are known to further exacerbate mental illnesses. As a result, many mentally ill people who also use opioids are at high risk of being stuck in a cycle of addiction.

Risk-Taking or Thrill-Seeking Actions

Individuals who habitually engage in risk-taking activities are more likely to become addicted to drugs than their more cautious counterparts. Drugs such as opioids tend to alter habits by causing changes in the brain. This can lower an individual's inhibition and make them daring and fearless. So, when people take drugs (*regularly*) in order to lower their inhibitions, they may end up becoming addicted to the thrill and become habitual users.

Stressful Circumstances

As human beings, we encounter challenging situations regularly in the course of our lives. Different people cope with stressful circumstances in their lives differently. While some may resort to confiding in their close friends and loved ones, others deal with stressful situations by indulging in opioid substances.

Career Path or Occupation

Research has shown that certain careers may increase the risk of drug use and addiction. For instance, in the arts and entertainment industry, there are a lot of famous actors, musicians, and other leading figures who have been in the news for illnesses or deaths due to drug use and abuse. This is not the only field that has such a high rate of addiction. Other career paths with the highest rates of drug and substance addiction include:

- Food and Hospitality Industry - According to reports by *Restaurant Business Online*, the food and hospitality industry has one of the highest rates of drug abuse, especially when it comes to illegal drugs. One in every five people working in this industry engages in the illicit use of drugs on a regular basis. In addition to taking illegal substances, employees also have a high rate of alcohol use as well as prescription opioids. The high prevalence of addiction is widely attributed to long working hours, and the pressure to perform at a very high level of customer service.

- Mining and Construction - The construction and mining industry is another career field that records very high numbers of drug abuse. According to the *Construction Executive Risk Management* magazine, 15 percent of construction workers regularly engage in the use of illicit drugs, while 18 percent frequently take alcohol. The high rate of drug and alcohol abuse in the construction industry often leads to serious injury, illnesses, and reduced productivity. Most of these employees hide their drug problems from their employers because they are afraid of losing their jobs. This usually exacerbates the problem and makes it even harder to mitigate.
- Business Management - The high-powered and fast-paced career of business management is known to be a great stress factor for professionals working in these fields. It is not surprising that a large number of business executives have been diagnosed with substance addiction. To deal with the stress experienced at the workplace, some managers often resort to the use of prescription opioids and other substances. This usually doesn't yield the desired results: Although the drugs provide temporary relief, the long term effects of prolonged use can be catastrophic. In light of this, numerous drug recovery programs now offer executive treatment plans that allow patients to continue working even as they undergo treatment. These programs also guarantee patients' privacy and confidentiality in order to ensure their professional lives are not negatively impacted.
- Healthcare Sector - It may seem ironic that the healthcare sector has a high prevalence of substance addiction, but many doctors and nurses are adversely affected by drug addiction. According to the National Council of State Boards of Nursing, career nurses who work in highly stressful situations are at high risk of drug use and abuse. Some of the nurses who are more susceptible to substance addiction

include those working in tasking environments such as emergency rooms, oncology centers, and psychiatric wards. The high rate of drug use and abuse in the healthcare sector can be attributed to the ease of access to these drugs. Most medical practitioners work in environments where prescription drugs can be easily acquired.

SIGNS OF ADDICTION

Drug abuse and addiction typically affect people differently depending on the factors that we highlighted in the previous section. There are, however, various symptoms that are common to drug users. These common symptoms may provide important insights on whether an individual has an addiction problem. These include:

Physical Dependence

Prolonged use of both legal and illegal opioids often leads to a build-up of tolerance. When this happens, a person may not be able to feel normal when they use their usual doses of a drug. As we all are aware, the build-up of tolerance may lead to addiction problems. As a result, the affected person may get used to drugs to a point where they are unable to function normally without them.

Signs of Outward Harm

Addiction to opioids often takes a toll on one's physical and mental health, as well as their habits. That is why individuals who are addicted to these drugs may expose themselves to hazardous situations in order to get their quick fix. They are also likely to neglect their social roles as well as personal health.

Compulsion to Use

The compulsion to use drugs is one of the most common signs of opioid addiction. Individuals who have used these drugs for prolonged periods may find it difficult to refrain from using them. Moreover, due to their high tolerance, they may start using larger amounts in order to experience the same effects, and they may find themselves using drugs for longer amounts of time.

Reduced Tolerance for Pain

Prescription opioids, as we discussed in the previous chapters, are designed to provide relief for mild and chronic pain. Doctors often recommend them for pain management in patients who are experiencing post-surgery pain or terminal illnesses. However, when these drugs are abused, they can interfere with one's neurol system, and make them have a reduced tolerance for pain. Such individuals may end up being addicted to opioids as they use them habitually to get rid of the pain.

Impaired Cognition

Prolonged use of opioid drugs may interfere with cognitive function in a number of ways. For instance, they may affect the brain's white matter, which is responsible for decision-making and memory. Long-term opioid users may manifest an inability to make decisions and respond to threatening situations appropriately.

Other signs of opioid dependency and addiction include:

- Constricted pupils
- Confusion
- Depression
- Constipation
- Runny nose
- Coordination problems
- Poor awareness of one's environment

Apart from the general symptoms of opioid abuse, there are several withdrawal symptoms that can help identify whether an individual is suffering from addiction. These include:

- Anxiety
- Uncontrollable shaking
- Sweating
- Intense cravings
- Vomiting
- Insomnia
- Abdominal discomfort

Unlike addictive drugs like marijuana, opioids generally have a very high risk of overdose. People who habitually use opioids, especially illegal ones like fentanyl, have a very high chance of overdosing. This is due to the fact that these outlawed drugs are often manufactured in combination with other dangerous substances such as cocaine and methamphetamines. It is not surprising, then, that most opioid-related overdoses are attributed to the use of illegal opioids.

An opioid overdose can cause serious damage to one's body organs, and may lead to death. In order to reverse the effects of the drug and to save lives, immediate treatment should be administered to opioid overdose patients. Here are some of the common signs and symptoms of opioid overdose:

- Constricted pupils
- Depressed breathing
- Drowsiness
- Confusion
- Drastic mood changes
- Uncontrolled vomiting
- Unconsciousness

In view of the life-threatening risks of opioid overdose, an individual who is suspected of having overdosed should be treated urgently to prevent fatality.

HOW OPIOID ADDICTION AFFECTS RELATIONSHIPS

Prolonged use of opioid drugs has the potential to completely alter an individual's temperament and actions. Consequently, this behavior can lead to social problems that deeply impact one's relationships in various ways, including:

Lies and Deception

One of the issues that people who are suffering from addiction struggle with is the need to maintain secrecy about their drug problem. This can be attributed to the stigma around drug addiction. Most opioid addicts are usually afraid of being judged by their friends, relatives, and society at large, due to their drug problem and they shame they may feel. They may also fear getting reported to authorities, losing their jobs or being victims of prejudice. As a result, they may go to extreme lengths to keep their habit a secret, and this may lead to turmoil in their relationships.

Loss of Trust

Due to their secretive lives and constant lying, people who struggle with opioid addiction are likely to experience trust issues in their relationships.

Furthermore, an opioid addict may prioritize their drug habit more than their partners, families, and friends. This can erode trust and cause turmoil in their relationships. Once this happens, it can be very challenging for the drug user to rebuild trust without first undergoing treatment for their drug problem.

Domestic Violence and Abuse

The pent up frustration and resentment that comes with addiction can easily blow over and manifest in angry outbursts leading to serious implications. Individuals who are addicted to drugs tend to be highly irritable, especially when they are experiencing withdrawal effects. This makes them easily triggered by even the most minute problems. Under these circumstances, a simple altercation can easily turn into a violent rage, which may have fatal consequences. Close family members such as the spouses and children of opioid addicts are at more risk of being victimized by their addicted family members.

Enabling Relationships

Sometimes, having a relationship with an individual who suffers from a drug problem can cloud one's judgment, and make them complicit in abetting the problem. They may end up making choices that enable their loved one's drug habit, without even being aware of it. Some examples of enabling habits include:

- Taking up the responsibilities of an individual who is addicted to opioids when they are unable to perform them.
- Downplaying or minimizing the negative consequences of a loved one's drug problem.
- Accepting blame for a loved one's drug addiction.
- Availing drugs to an addicted individual when they experience withdrawal symptoms.
- Proving financial assistance to addicted individuals in order to fund their substance use and abuse.

It is very easy for an individual to miss the thin line between helping a struggling loved one and abetting their drug habit. This is why most people often end up exacerbating their loved one's addiction despite their best intentions. Often, these people act with good intentions without realizing that they are actually endangering the lives of addicted individuals.

Co-Dependent Relationships

Opioid addiction often results in co-dependent relationships, which are toxic to both parties. A codependent partner who is in a relationship with an opioid addict may be suffering from the consequences of their loved one's addiction, while at the same time, strongly holding a sense of duty towards them. They may feel that it is their responsibility to take care of their loved one and help them overcome their addiction. They may even enjoy serving in the role of caregiver to their loved ones.

While there is nothing inherently wrong about wanting to care for a drug addict, being too self-sacrificing can seriously affect one's physical and mental health, especially if the outcome expected is not forthcoming. Even though it's very noble to be concerned about a struggling loved one, take care not to be at the center of the addiction in their lives. In doing so, you will be able to remain grounded and rational even as you contend with the dynamic nature of the relationship with your addicted loved one.

As we come to the conclusion of the first half of this book, let us recap some of the most important takeaways from this chapter.

- Several models can be used to map the cause and progression of addiction. These include: Automatic Processing Theories; reflective Choice theories; Goal-Oriented Theories; and Integrative theories.
- An individual's risk of opioid addiction is influenced by a number of internal and external factors including poverty, unemployment, exposure to high-risk individuals and environments, previous history of substance abuse, mental illness and many others.
- Prolonged opioid use can significantly alter a person's habits and increase their risk of dependency and addiction. Consequently, this increases their chances of overdosing on these drugs, which can prove fatal.
- Opioid addiction can lead to loss of trust in relationships and increase the likelihood of domestic violence. This can

significantly damage one's social life and contribute to further health problems such as depression.

At this point, I am certain that you now have a thorough understanding of the opioid problem, what causes addiction and the manner in which it presents in individuals. In the next and final half of this book, we are going to turn our attention to healing and discussing the strategies that can be applied to help an individual overcome opioid addiction. Some of the key topics that will be addressed in the coming chapters include: how to use prescription opioids safely and responsibly; how to incorporate medicines in the treatment of opioid addiction and the importance of seeking the help of others when fighting opioid addiction. Finally, we shall delve into non-drug and natural treatments that are available for preventing opioid addiction.

5

IF YOU NEED THEM, USE THEM RESPONSIBLY

Despite their addictive nature, there are moments when the use of opioid drugs may be necessary. For instance, if you are suffering from chronic pain due to injury, terminal illness or after surgery, your doctor may recommend an opioid medication to help manage the pain. If no other treatment is available, the use of prescription opioids might be the only viable option left. In light of the risks and dangers involved in opioid use, it is vital to take the necessary precautions to ensure that your health is not jeopardized. Having the right information about the effects of opioids, both positive and negative, can empower you to use these drugs responsibly if you require them for your pain-management needs.

Let us now turn our attention to some of the practices you need to cultivate in order to ensure you are using prescription opioids in the right manner. As you read this chapter, try to identify the key areas where you may need to improve when medicating with prescription opioids.

Stick to the Prescription

While prescription opioids are commonly prescribed to patients suffering from chronic pain, many individuals often fail to adhere to the instructions given by their doctors. Though many people tend to assume that failure to stick to the prescription is harmless, studies have shown that this practice can put one's health in serious jeopardy.

There are several reasons why many patients fail to adhere to the prescriptions instructions outlined by their physician. Some do so due to a lack of understanding of the directions given; some people fail to stick to the prescription due to forgetfulness. Individuals who are taking several medications at once are likely to forget the exact prescription of certain drugs. Unpleasant effects from the medication may also discourage an individual from using them in the right amounts. This is undoubtedly true with opioid medications, which are commonly known to produce serious side effects as we have discussed in the previous chapter.

The high cost of prescription opioids may also prevent some individuals from using the drugs as recommended. Patients who are unable to afford the drugs on a regular basis may opt to take fewer doses than what's prescribed to make the prescription last longer.

Regardless of one's motive for not adhering to the recommended prescription, not following directions can be very harmful and detrimental to one's health. Failure to stick to the required doses may cause the treatment to stall, and make the drug ineffective. This could cause the patient's condition to deteriorate so rapidly that they may end up being hospitalized. In more extreme cases, failure to take the right dosage may lead to fatality.

In light of these risks, sticking to the recommended prescription is very important especially when taking opioid medications. How can you ensure that you are following the regimen outlined by your doctor? Here are some of tips that can help you stick to your prescription:

- Schedule a specific time for taking your medication every day.
- Combine the time you take your medication with another activity such as preparing for bedtime, brushing your teeth, etc.
- Keep track of your medication using a 'calendar.' Make sure you keep a record of the pills you take on a daily basis.
- When traveling, make sure you bring enough pills to last several extra days in case your return is delayed.
- Use a pill container to organize the drugs according to the time of day that you are supposed to take them, e.g., breakfast, lunch, after dinner, etc.

Make Sure You Know the Risks

Before starting any prescription opioid regimen, it is essential to be informed of the risk factors involved. Whereas opioid drugs are very effective when it comes to pain management, there are numerous risks that they may pose to the patients who take them. Apart from the negative side effects that we highlighted in the previous chapters, some of these drugs have interactions with other medications, herbs, and food, which may result in morbidity and mortality.

The interaction of prescription opioids with other drugs can be classified as either pharmacodynamic or pharmacokinetic. The former refers to interactions in which the drugs influence each other's effects directly. In such a case, when the two drugs are administered concurrently, the concentration-response of one or both of the drugs is altered without any change in the pharmacokinetics of the object drug.

Pharmacodynamic drug-drug interactions can be either additive, synergistic or antagonistic. An additive interaction is a situation whereby the effect of the two substances is equal to the sum of the effect of the two drugs taken separately, whereas in a synergistic interaction the effect of two drugs when used together is greater than the sum of their separate effect at the same doses. Conversely, an antagonistic interaction is a situation where the effect of two drugs is less than the sum of the effect of the two drugs when taken separately.

On the other hand, a pharmacokinetic drug-drug interaction happens when one drug (a precipitant) interferes in the absorption, distribution, metabolism, and excretion of the other drug (the object). This type of interaction can lead to a reduction in the concentration of an opioid drug, thereby making it less therapeutic and effective.

The interaction of prescription opioids with other medications may also have adverse effects on persons with pre-existing medical conditions. The pharmacodynamic interactions of opioids may, for instance, increase the risk of respiratory depression in patients who have cardiovascular or cerebrovascular conditions. Patients who have brain injuries, dementia or psychiatric illnesses are also at higher risk of cognitive impairment when exposed to opioid medications.

Likewise, individuals who have a history of substance abuse are more likely to develop dependence and addiction to prescription opioids compared with those who have never used drugs.

Questions to Ask your Doctor

In order to use prescription opioids responsibly, it is essential to be sufficiently informed about these drugs. If you intend to use these drugs to manage your medical condition, there are several questions you may ask your doctor in order to receive clarification on their suitability to your condition. These questions include:

i) Why was I prescribed opioids and are they the best option for me?

You may be well aware by now that prescription opioids are generally used as pain-relief medications. Doctors often recommend these drugs to patients who are suffering from chronic pain due to physical injury, terminal illness, and recent surgery. If you are experiencing pain due to any of these reasons, there is a chance that your doctor may prescribe an opioid drug to help you cope with the pain.

Since these drugs often come with a whole slew of side effects, you should make sure you understand these possible side effects that you may have to deal with when medicating on opioids. If you are in chronic pain, prescription opioids may be the only option you have despite the unpleasant side effects that may accompany their use. On the other hand, if your pain is mild, there are various non-drug options that may be more appropriate and safer to use.

Before you start taking these drugs, your doctor should explain why they are prescribing them, and they should offer alternatives in case the drugs fail to deliver desired results, based on your situation.

ii) Will opioids cause side effects that could affect the quality of my life?

Prescription opioids are very powerful and potent drugs that produce a wide array of side effects. Apart from the physical effects such as respiratory distress, sweating, vomiting, and abdominal pains, opioid use may also cause long-lasting cognitive changes. Individuals who use these drugs for prolonged periods of time may experience significant mood changes, increased tolerance, dependence, and possible addiction. All of these effects have serious implications on a user's overall health and wellbeing.

Before starting out on prescription opioids, it is important to be aware of both the short-term and long-term effects that these drugs may have on your health.

iii) Should I be concerned about starting opioids/stopping them?

Prolonged use of opioid medications is known to cause tolerance build-up, which may lead to dependency. Even individuals who use these drugs as prescribed by a doctor may end up developing a high tolerance for them. This can reduce the effectiveness of the medication and necessitate an increase in dosage. As a result, people who regularly use these drugs may end up becoming hooked on them. This is obviously a serious concern to take into account when making the decision on whether or not to use these drugs.

In cases where addiction has set in, it may be very difficult to abstain from prescription opioids due to the withdrawal symptoms that they are likely to experience. Furthermore, the long-term use of prescription opioids for pain management can significantly reduce one's tolerance for pain. As a result, an individual may end up using the drugs perpetually.

iv) What are other pain management treatments?

The fact that you may be experiencing chronic pain does not automatically mean that prescription opioids are the solution. Whereas these drugs can be highly effective in providing pain relief, they also come with a lot of unpleasant side-effects, which might be more detrimental to your health. If possible, try to explore other treatment methods that may be more suitable for your condition before deciding whether or not to use opioids.

There are various non-pharmacological therapies that can be used to manage chronic pain. These include treatments such as acupuncture, relaxation techniques, massage therapy, and gel packs. Being aware of the various non-drug therapies available can help you make the right choice when deciding on the safest pain management treatment to apply.

v) Could a physician who specializes in pain management help me?

Having a specialized therapist can be invaluable when it comes to chronic pain management. A qualified specialist can evaluate your condition and devise the right treatment strategy for your situation. Depending on your health status, they may recommend using opioids, non-drug treatments or a combination of both.

Keep them Out of the Reach of the People Living around You.

One of the factors that contribute to the misuse and abuse of prescription drugs is the practice of sharing. Many individuals who have prescriptions of these drugs often feel inclined to share with their friends or relatives. This practice can have serious implications for all individuals involved, due to a number of reasons.

Sharing your prescription opioids with others reduces your consignment, and may shorten your dosage. This can force you to cut down on the recommended prescription. Consequently, this can jeopardize the effectiveness of the medication and cause the entire treatment to fail.

The practice can also put your close relatives and friends at serious risk. As we have reiterated several times over the course of this book, opioids are very potent drugs that must be consumed under the recommendations of a qualified medical professional. By using these drugs without a prescription, an individual risks developing tolerance, dependence and addiction, which can be very difficult to treat.

For this reason, it is important to ensure that you use the drugs responsibly. Do not share them with anyone, and always store your drugs safely to prevent them from falling into the wrong hands, e.g. young children.

Know When It's Time to Stop

One of the hardest things about using prescription opioids is knowing when it is time to stop using them, and how to make that transition. Opioids are naturally addictive, partly due to the pleasant symptoms they induce. In addition to their pain-relieving properties, prescription opioids often generate feelings of sedation and euphoria when ingested. That's why when an individual becomes too accustomed to this feeling, it may be very difficult for them to quit using these drugs, even when the original purpose of using them has already been achieved.

In order to use these drugs responsibly, you need to realize when the drugs have served their purpose, and you no longer need them. Your physician or anesthesiologist can help you come off these drugs by doing the following:

- Individualizing your tapering plan to minimize the effects of your withdrawal symptoms
- Constantly monitoring your withdrawal effects
- Adjusting the rate and duration of your tapering process appropriately, depending on the withdrawal effects that you are experiencing
- Recommending additional sources of support that can help you give up the drugs safely

Watch out for Withdrawal Symptoms

When opioids are used for extended periods of time, they may lead to a condition known as opioid withdrawal syndrome. This arises out of drug dependency, and is characterized by the inability of an individual to function normally without using the opioids. The rate at which individuals develop dependency varies from person to person. Once they have become dependent on these drugs, it can be very difficult for them to function without taking them.

If you are trying to quit using opioids, you need to realize that it will take some time for the body to shed off its addiction to the drugs and begin functioning normally again. That's why it is crucial to pay close attention to the symptoms that are manifesting, as you cut down on and eventually quit opioid use.

Some of the early stage withdrawal symptoms that you need to keep an eye on include:

- Insomnia
- Muscle aches and pains
- Sweating
- Nausea
- Vomiting
- Diarrhea

In addition to these short-term symptoms, there are several long-term withdrawal symptoms that you may experience when you first try to quit opioid use. These include:

- Abdominal cramping
- Increased heart rate
- Uncontrollable shaking
- Dilated pupils

Although these withdrawal symptoms are not life-threatening, they can be very uncomfortable and painful to endure when you are trying to give up on opioid use. These symptoms are key indicators of how your body is coping with the absence of opioids. By observing these symptoms, your anesthesiologist can be able to determine the right dose for you at every stage, during the process of giving up on opioids.

TRY SEEKING ALTERNATIVE PAIN RELIEF PRACTICES

Dealing with constant chronic pain can be challenging for anyone. Most people end up seeking prescription opioids for their pain-relieving properties. There are, though, several alternative treatments that can be used to alleviate chronic pain. These non-drug options are not only effective, but also desirable, since they do not produce adverse side effects that are commonly associated with prescription opioids. Some of the alternative non-pharmacological treatments that you can opt for include:

Combined Therapy

In most cases, opioids by themselves are not very useful when it comes to pain management; they may cause negative side effects which may jeopardize the treatment. As a result, many physicians often recommend combined therapy involving both the use of opioids and non-drug treatments to manage chronic pain. Since minimal amounts of opioids are used in combined therapy, the risk of developing tolerance and dependence is significantly low.

Non-Drug Therapies

In cases where opioids are ineffective or counterproductive to managing pain, patients can find relief with the help of non-drug therapies. Some of the most common non-drug treatments that may be recommended include acupuncture, meditation, biofeedback, and massage therapy. These treatments are very safe, and can be applied with little to no adverse side effects. If you are struggling with chronic pain, it is vital to seek help from an expert who will recommend the best non-drug therapy for you.

Injections or Implants

In case you are experiencing neuropathic pain or muscle spasms, getting a local anesthetic injection may be a sufficient alternative to short-circuit the pain. Similarly, if you are suffering from chronic pain in your arms, back, and legs, your physician may recommend getting a spinal cord stimulation procedure. This typically involves having a device implanted in a patient's back to block pain by transmitting electric pulses to the spinal cord and nerves. These alternative treatments can help you manage chronic pain much more effectively while protecting you from the numerous risks that are involved in pharmacological therapies.

The responsible use of opioid drugs is essential when it comes to pain-management therapy using these drugs. Failure to observe the recommended precautions can put one at risk of significant physical and mental health problems. Here are the main takeaways on the practices that you should always uphold when using prescription opioids to relieve pain:

- Always use the medication in the right doses.
- Ensure that you are well informed on the risks that are involved with opioid use before you start using these drugs.
- Refrain from sharing your prescription opioids with your friends and family members.
- Always ensure that your drugs are stored safely away from the reach of children and other susceptible individuals.
- Look out for any withdrawal symptoms that you may be experiencing as you try to cut down or completely stop taking these drugs. Make sure to inform your doctor about these so that they can recommend the appropriate treatment for your condition.
- Seek non-drug therapies to help you manage your pain safely.

6

MEDICATION AS TREATMENT

While prescription opioids are very useful as pain-relief medication, the personal price of using them may at times be too high to bear. Once an individual starts using opioid drugs, their tolerance often builds up gradually until they are unable to operate normally without consuming high doses of the drug.

Persons that have used prescription opioids for long periods of time are likely to be stuck in a cycle of addiction unless they receive the right treatment and support. The treatment for addiction typically includes short term therapy to manage withdrawal symptoms, long-term treatment of withdrawal symptoms, and overdose treatment. The type of treatment administered often depends on the severity of the problem.

SHORT-TERM TREATMENT OF WITHDRAWAL SYMPTOMS

Opioid dependence is usually accompanied by withdrawal symptoms that range from mild to severe. Treatment for these symptoms is generally determined by their severity and duration. In general, the withdrawal symptoms of most opioids usually kick in 6 to 12 hours after use, and may last for up to 5 days. While these symptoms are not life-threatening, they can be very unpleasant. That is why individuals who are suffering from withdrawal symptoms are likely to relapse back to active drug use.

To break the cycle of addiction, it is essential for victims of opioid use disorder to receive immediate treatment. There are various indicators that influence the onset and duration of opioid effects. These include:

- If the drug is used intermittently, withdrawal effects are unlikely to appear
- High intake of prescription opioids for longer durations of time raises the risk of withdrawal effects
- Short-acting opioids and slowly injected morphine have a more rapid onset and shorter withdrawal duration
- Longer-acting opioids such as methadone have a slower onset but more lasting withdrawal symptoms

Medications such as buprenorphine and methadone have been approved by the FDA for short term treatment of opioid withdrawal symptoms. These drugs must be administered under the guidance of a qualified medical practitioner or physician.

LONG-TERM MAINTENANCE TREATMENT

Opioid dependence and addiction are highly complex health conditions that require long-term treatment and management. Early treatment can help an individual regain their physical and psychological health, thus enabling them to become functional and productive members of society.

The aim of long-term maintenance treatment is to successfully rehabilitate individuals who are struggling with opioid addiction, reduce their dependence on these drugs, and eliminate the risk of overdose.

Since no single treatment is effective for treating all individuals who suffer from opioid addiction, therapy usually combines several treatments, including medication and behavioral therapy.

The FDA has approved various medications for opioid addiction treatment. These include the mu-opioid agonists methadone and buprenorphine or the opioid antagonist, naltrexone. Let us briefly discuss some of these pharmacological agents and how they work in relation to opioid addiction treatment.

Naltrexone

Naltrexone is an opioid antagonist drug that is commonly used to treat patients who suffer from addiction to opiate drugs like morphine, codeine, and heroin. The drug can also be used to treat individuals who are addicted to alcohol and recovering addicts to prevent a relapse.

Naltrexone generally works by blocking the effects of opioid drugs such as euphoria, pain relief, and sedation. Since most people tend to get hooked on opioids to experience these effects, the use of naltrexone treats addiction by eliminating the need or desire to use opioids.

This drug is typically administered orally, and can be consumed with or without food. It is also important for this treatment to be supervised by a professional physician so that they can keep track of the progress and note any effects that may be manifesting (in the early stages) in the patient.

Not all people, however, are allowed to take this drug. You are advised to avoid naltrexone if:

- You are still using other prescription opioids such as morphine, heroin, and methadone
- You experience extreme allergic reactions after taking the drug

- You are experiencing withdrawal symptoms from using other drugs or alcohol
- You have used any other opioid medication in the past 10 days

In order to ensure the safe use of this drug, you should inform your doctor if you have the following conditions:

- Liver disease
- Kidney disease
- Blood clot
- Respiratory illnesses

Using opioid medications while on naltrexone may induce withdrawal symptoms. Some of the most common side effects of using this drug include:

- Nausea and vomiting
- Diarrhea
- Mood changes
- Hallucination
- Confusion
- Depression
- Dizziness
- Insomnia

These symptoms are not life-threatening, and may taper off after a few days. If you do experience adverse effects, you should inform your doctor immediately. You should also refrain from sharing this medicine with others and store it safely away from the reach of children.

Buprenorphine

Buprenorphine is a weak partial mu-opioid receptor agonist used as an alternative medication for treating severe opioid addiction. It usually helps in fighting addiction by preventing the withdrawal symptoms resulting from halting the use of opioids. The drug is often used in combination with counseling sessions to provide a holistic treatment for opioid addiction.

Buprenorphine is usually administered orally - put it under the tongue and allow it to dissolve completely. It is often administered together with Naloxone to prevent misuse of the medication. For best results, buprenorphine should be given to a patient as soon as the first signs of withdrawal take effect. If the drug is administered soon after one has taken other opioid medications, withdrawal effects may ensue.

If one stops taking buprenorphine sooner than required, one may also experience adverse withdrawal effects including nausea, runny nose, diarrhea, and insomnia. For this reason, doctors are usually advised to slowly lower the dose administered to patients in order to prevent these symptoms.

Methadone

Methadone is an opioid drug that is used to relieve chronic pain in patients who need medication for pain management but cannot be treated by other drugs. This medication is also commonly used to prevent withdrawal symptoms in patients who are trying to recover from opioid addiction.

The drug works by blocking the effects of opioid medications such as heroin, codeine, and hydrocodone. Since it produces similar effects to other prescription opioids, methadone is commonly used as part of replacement therapy. It can also be combined with counseling and non-pharmacological therapies to maximize the effectiveness of the treatment.

Methadone comes in a variety of forms including tablets, powder, and liquid solutions. Although the drug is legal, and widely available in most pharmacies, one needs a doctor's prescription to obtain it. In most cases of opioid addiction, doctors recommend that methadone is used for at least a year during the recovery period. Once it is time to stop using the drug, your doctor will slowly reduce your dose of the drug to prevent withdrawal symptoms.

Some of the common side effects associated with this drug include:

- Restlessness
- Vomiting
- Respiratory depression
- Itchy skin
- Loss of appetite
- Abdominal discomfort
- Headache
- Mood changes

These symptoms are typically mild, and tend to dissipate after a few days. In some cases, severe symptoms may be experienced by individuals who are using methadone to treat opioid addiction. Some of the adverse side effects of using this drug may include:

- Fainting
- Swollen lips, tongue or face
- Faster heartbeat
- Seizures
- Drowsiness
- Trouble swallowing

LAAM (levomethadyl acetate)

LAAM is a synthetic opioid drug that works in a manner similar to methadone. This medication is usually administered to opioid-dependent individuals to block the effects of other opioid medications, thereby eliminating the craving for these drugs.

Just like methadone, LAAM has been approved by the FDA for treating opioid addiction. The effects of this drug are usually longer lasting compared to methadone. This makes it possible for LAAM to be taken on alternate days, unlike methadone which must be taken daily.

Like most opioid agonists, LAAM can cause physical dependence when used for prolonged periods. As a result, doctors often reduce the dosage gradually to prevent withdrawal symptoms from manifesting.

Some of the common side effects that are associated with this drug include:

- Muscle and joint pain
- Insomnia
- Constipation
- Nervousness
- Drowsiness
- Dizziness
- Poor concentration

LAAM should not be taken by patients who are using other prescription opioids, alcohol, benzodiazepines, and antidepressants. The drug is also not recommended for use during pregnancy as it can have adverse effects on the developing fetus.

Naloxone

Naloxone is an opioid antagonist drug that is used to block or reverse the effects of opioid medications including loss of consciousness, drowsiness, and slow breathing. This drug is commonly administered as an injection, especially in case of emergencies such as opioid overdose. Similarly, naloxone is used to diagnose whether an individual has overdosed on opioids.

There are various scenarios where the use of this drug is not recommended. These include:

- Pregnancy
- If one is taking alcohol or any other opioid drug
- If the individual is allergic to the drug
- If one is suffering from chronic conditions such as heart disease, liver disease, and respiratory illnesses
- If one is breastfeeding

Since naloxone works by reversing the effects of opioid medications, withdrawal symptoms may be experienced by persons using this drug. Some of the common side effects of this antagonist opioid include:

- Diarrhea
- Nausea and vomiting
- Stomach pain
- Fever
- Body aches
- Nervousness
- Irritability
- Runny nose

Naloxone is known to interact with other prescription and over-the-counter drugs, vitamins, and herbal products. Nevertheless, the drug is often used to treat opioid-related drug overdoses where it is administered as an emergency treatment. In such a scenario, it may not be possible to inform your doctor about your medical history, so the chances of developing complications are very high.

For this reason, if you are a friend or relative of the drug addict, it is important to provide any relevant information on the history of the patient that would help medical professionals to facilitate the recovery process.

TREATMENT OF OVERDOSE

People who use opioid medications either medically or recreationally are at very high risk of overdosing on these drugs. This risk is particularly greater for individuals who use illicit synthetic opioids like fentanyl. The overdose can lead to slowed breathing that can cause significant brain damage, organ failure, and even death. In light of this, immediate care should be administered to an overdose victim to save their lives, and prevent serious damage to their health.

Opioid overdose happens when an individual has excessive stimulation of the opiate pathway. This can cause respiratory depression and possibly lead to death. Some of the common causes of opioid overdose include:

- Therapeutic drug error
- Intentional overdose
- Unintentional overdose
- Complications related to opioid abuse

Possible signs and symptoms of an opioid overdose include:

- Slow /difficulty in breathing
- Unconsciousness
- Unresponsiveness to outside stimulus
- Vomiting
- Pale face and body
- Slow heartbeat
- Choking sounds

Initial treatment for an opioid overdose is usually administered depending on the vital signs. For instance, if a patient is comatose due to opioid overdose and is not breathing, they should first be provided with airway control before any further treatment is administered. An endotracheal intubation is often conducted to protect their airways. Thereafter, naloxone may be administered to reverse the effects of respiratory depression. It should be noted, however, that naloxone can also cause aggression or agitation, and must be administered in minimal amounts depending on a patient's response.

Once a patient has been provided with the first line of treatment at the scene of the overdose, they should be transferred to the emergency department of a hospital. If the patient has already received treatment for respiratory distress, the doctors should check for any signs of occult trauma to the cervical spine. In some cases, when patients who are suspected of having overdosed on opioids are transferred to the emergency room, they may have their blood glucose levels drawn.

Emergency treatment typically begins with supportive care, including respiratory assistance through CPR and removal of the opioid agent in the case of the drug having been delivered using a patch. If the doctor suspects an opioid overdose, the antagonist drug naloxone should be administered immediately either intravenously, subcutaneously or intramuscularly.

When administered intravenously, naloxone takes effect after a few minutes. A second dose may be given after 2 to 3 minutes. When naloxone is administered intramuscularly or subcutaneously, the onset action may take up to 10 minutes. Once the overdosed patient is awake, the dose of naloxone should be disconnected. In patients who overdose on opioids such as methadone and heroin, larger doses of naloxone should be administered.

Sometimes, naloxone is used in combination with buprenorphine to treat opioid overdose. The advantage of this drug combination is that it can reduce withdrawal symptoms for up to 36 hours.

Most patients who overdose on opioids and are treated with naloxone may be admitted to an emergency facility for monitoring for about 12 to 36 hours. Likewise, patients who require more than one dose of naloxone to reverse their overdose are also admitted for observation. Due to the risk of respiratory depression in emergency overdoses, many doctors are increasingly promoting take-home naloxone for high-risk opioid users.

Once a patient has been treated successfully for an opioid overdose, they should continually be provided with psychological counseling and therapy to help them overcome their opioid use, and avoid a relapse.

Although opioid addiction and overdose can be very destructive and life-threatening, it is possible for an individual to be treated successfully as long as they are diagnosed early and provided with immediate medical assistance.

As we come to the end of this chapter, here are the most important points to remember:

- There are several drugs that have been approved for opioid addiction treatment by the FDA. These include buprenorphine, naloxone, naltrexone, methadone and levomethadyl acetate (LAAM)
- Opioid antagonists should be administered to patients immediately to reverse the effects of opioid drugs and ease respiratory distress
- Individuals who are recovering from opioid addiction should reduce their dose of antagonist drugs gradually in order to reduce withdrawal effects.
- Opioid overdose patients may be hospitalized or treated outpatient depending on the severity of their symptoms once emergency care has been administered.

SEEK THE HELP OF OTHERS

In our society, there is a widely held perception that addiction is a personal problem that arises out of weakness of character or from making poor life choices. The idea that substance addiction is an actual illness that affects the physical and psychological balance of a person is still inconceivable to many people. As a result of this common misconception, many people tend to treat individuals who are struggling with addiction as outcasts who should be isolated from others lest they influence them negatively. This kind of response to addiction, however, usually does more harm than good. It is vital that we remind ourselves that those who suffer from addiction are human beings who deserve the care and protection of society just like everyone else. It is especially important that they are supported so that they can recover fully from addiction and become productive members of society.

In this section, we will highlight the role that family members, friends, and society all play in the fight against opioid addiction. If you are struggling with addiction yourself, this chapter will show you the importance of seeking the help of others to aid your recovery and the ways in which you can do that.

Clinical Psychology of Addiction

While opioid addiction is commonly regarded as a physical illness due to the physical symptoms that it manifests, this problem is also psychological to a great extent. Early on, we discussed the cognitive ramifications of addiction, and saw how the problem of opioid dependence and addiction can alter one's mood and cause an imbalance in mental states. Nevertheless, the disease of opioid addiction can also be triggered by several psychological issues. In order for the right treatment to be administered, it is important to understand the psychological aspect of addiction.

Although opioid addiction is mainly a result of various modifications in a person's body, recovery necessitates that those who are affected by this problem apply significant changes in their relationship with these drugs. Like most human actions, opioid addiction is a habit that is learned. Since psychology is the study of human practices, exploring the psychological makeup of opioid addicts can provide us with important insights into this condition and subsequently guide the decision toward the right approach to treatment.

Another psychological factor that may cause or perpetuate the problem of addiction is people's beliefs and thoughts. It is no secret that our own actions tend to be influenced by our thoughts and beliefs. This means an individual's beliefs about opioid addiction may determine whether or not they are able to overcome this disease. For instance, a person who believes they can't recover from opioid addiction is unlikely to put in the effort required to kick the habit. On the contrary, an individual who considers opioid addiction as a disease that can be treated is likely to be motivated to follow through on treatment, and exert themselves fully in trying to overcome this challenge.

Likewise, a person's level of developmental maturity may also influence whether or not they are able to overcome the problem of addiction. If an individual routinely acts according to every craving, desire or whim without exercising critical thinking, they are likely to become addicted to opioids due to low developmental maturity. The person may end up getting hooked on drugs simply because they act out of impulse without thinking about the ramifications of their actions.

Individuals who manifest opioid addiction as a result of these psychological comorbidities can be helped to overcome this disease through psychotherapy.

Drug Addiction and Mental Health Diagnosis

Numerous studies conducted over the past couple of years have established a link between drug addiction and mental health. It is estimated that at least 8.2 million adults who were suffering from addiction had concurrent mental illness diagnoses. Even more surprising is the fact that only 48 percent of these people received treatment for either their drug problem or mental illness. This means more than half of these respondents did not receive treatment for either of these conditions.

This shortage of treatment for dual diagnoses of addiction and mental illness can be attributed to the fact that very few rehabilitation programs are equipped to deal with these cases. As a result, most people who seek therapy for their opioid addiction and mental illnesses are not able to receive the treatment they require. This is undoubtedly a very unfortunate situation, considering the fact that individuals with concurrent disorders are at greater risk of relapsing.

Comprehensive treatment and care can significantly reduce the risk of relapse in individuals who are recovering from opioid addiction. In order for this to happen, there has to be a paradigm shift in which the problem of addiction is treated as a mental illness instead of a criminal activity or irresponsible behavior.

Opioid addiction is characterized as a mental illness because it causes significant changes in the brain, which can alter one's mood and actions in extreme ways. Once an individual becomes dependent on these substances, their ability to control their impulses and cravings is compromised. Consequently, an opioid addict may find it difficult to stop using these substances, even when they are aware of the dangers that they expose themselves to. This compulsive behavior is quite similar to the manner in which mentally ill individuals act.

How exactly should the treatment of addiction be approached when dealing with individuals who are also diagnosed with mental illness? Studies have shown that among patients with moderate to severe dual diagnoses disorders, the chances for successful treatment are higher when the addiction treatment is supplemented with targeted psychological therapies. Like most other mental health illnesses, opioid addiction often requires long-term treatment and maintenance. This is contrary to the commonly held belief that only will power is required in order to kick a drug habit.

The connection between mental health and drug abuse is not always as clear-cut as some may be inclined to think. Whereas opioid addiction can give rise to mental health problems, there are certain scenarios where the addiction problem itself arises out of poor mechanisms of coping with mental illness. For instance, some individuals may use drugs like morphine and heroin as a means of self-medicating their mental illnesses such as depression and anxiety. These strategies, however, often lead to catastrophic outcomes and may exacerbate the problem.

There are several ways in which the symptoms of mental illness and opioid addiction can trigger each other. These include:

- Chronic use of opioids can increase an individual's risk of being a victim of violent crime or rape, which may lead to mental health problems like PTSD and depression.
- Bad decisions made under the influence of opioid drugs can make one susceptible to criminal activities, which may get them in trouble and contribute to anxiety.

When it comes to dual diagnosis disorders, the treatment approach should encompass both addiction treatment as well as mental health therapies. Without a comprehensive treatment plan for dual diagnosis, the risk of patients relapsing to drug use is very high. If one's mental health symptoms are not fully treated, it can be very difficult for a person to remain sober and possibly provide an incentive for them to use opioids to self-medicate. Conversely, if their opioid addiction symptoms are not addressed through a comprehensive treatment model, the individual can spiral deeper into addiction, and consequently develop more serious mental health conditions.

DIFFERENT TREATMENT APPROACHES FOR DRUG ADDICTION

Although addiction is a treatable condition, it is also a very chronic problem that requires a multi-layered approach. Individuals who have developed a dependency on drugs cannot simply quit using drugs for a few days and be completely cured. Most patients of opioid addiction typically require long-term treatment and care in order to successfully overcome the habit. That is why treatment for opioid addiction should be focussed on helping individuals to stop using drugs in the short-term, become drug-free for the long-term, and return to being productive members of society.

There are various principles that should form the foundation of any addiction treatment. These include acknowledging that:

- Addiction is a complex disease, with the potential of completely altering a person's way of life.
- No single kind of treatment is suitable for everyone.
- Individuals who are struggling with addiction need to be able to access treatment quickly.
- In order for treatment to be effective, it needs to address all the patient's needs, not just their drug use.

- Counseling and behavioral therapies are essential in order for treatment to be effective.
- Medication is an integral part of opioid dependence and addiction treatment.
- Treatment programs should be reviewed regularly and customized to suit the ever-changing needs of the patient.
- Opioid addiction treatment should also address the mental health of the patient.
- The patients' drug use should be monitored constantly throughout the duration of treatment.
- Treatment need not be voluntary.

There are various treatment approaches that can be used to treat opioid addiction successfully. These include:

Cognitive-Behavioral Therapy (CBT)

This is a form of mental health counseling that is widely used in addiction treatment today. This psychological counseling is designed to help addicts find connections between their thoughts, emotions, and actions. This counseling increases their awareness of themselves and allows them to foster positive habits to overcome dependence.

In addition to treating addiction, CBT can be very effective when it comes to managing various mental illnesses including, bipolar disorder, obsessive-compulsive disorder, depression, and post-traumatic stress disorder.

How exactly does this therapy work? The goal of CBT is to help patients become more aware that not all of their thoughts, feelings, and actions are rational or logical. Through CBT, individuals who struggle with opioid addiction are able to develop a wider perspective on their illness and see the way in which past experiences and environmental factors influence their drug problem.

Cognitive-behavioral therapists assist individuals who are recovering from addiction to identify negative automatic thoughts that make them susceptible to opioid use. By continually revisiting painful thoughts and memories which they harbor within them, recovering addicts are able to reduce the pain caused by these painful thoughts and memories. The result is help to eliminate urges and impulses that may predispose them to opioid use. They are also able to learn positive practices, which can replace their addictive tendencies.

CBT allows opioid-dependent individuals to kick their addiction by:

- Helping overcome negative thoughts and beliefs which make them likely to use drugs.
- Training on how to communicate better with their friends and colleagues.
- Providing self-help techniques and tools which can help to improve their mood.

The therapy also trains opioid-dependent individuals to become aware of triggers that spark opioid cravings. Some of the skills that CBT aims to teach opioid-dependent individuals include:

- Recognition - This is the ability to identify the circumstances or situations that trigger the urge to use drugs. Being able to pick on the situations that make you susceptible to drug use is necessary in order to remove you from the triggering situations or handle it more positively.
- Avoidance - Patients are trained on how to remove themselves from situations that trigger the impulse to take opioid drugs.
- Coping - CBT provides patients with techniques and tools that can address the underlying thoughts and emotions, which often lead to drug abuse.

CBT can be administered in a therapist's office, remotely at home, in the form of individual therapy sessions or group therapy meetings where recovering opioid addicts can interact with and share their stories with others.

Twelve-Step Approaches

This treatment approach involves group meetings where individuals who are struggling with addiction can share their experiences with each other and find solidarity, comfort, and hope. These support meetings are very important since they provide opioid-dependent individuals with a safe and non-judgmental space to share their stories.

Addiction stigma is still very rampant in our society, and many people have a very disparaging attitude towards people who are addicted to drugs. This may discourage struggling drug addicts from seeking treatment. Through the twelve-step approach, the opioid-dependent patients are able to receive the treatment and support they need to go through rehabilitation and recover from their illness.

This strategy is based on the premise that people can help each other to achieve and maintain abstinence from opioid drugs. There are several emotional and mental transformative tools and techniques that the twelve-step approach aims to impart to opioid-dependent patients. These include:

- The ability to recognize their addiction problem as an illness.
- The awareness of addiction as a problem that exists, and one that requires outer intervention and aid.
- The practice of self-observation to become aware of the habits that gave rise to the addiction problem.
- Techniques to help one develop self-restraint and confidence in their ability to recover from addiction.
- Developing self-acceptance and the ability to overcome negative coping mechanisms.

- Cultivating compassion towards others who struggle with addiction and their affected families.
- Tools that foster continual recovery in the long run.

With the help of these tools and strategies, individuals are empowered to change habits that enable their opioid addiction and learn positive ones that can help them recover. Here are the twelve steps that are envisioned in this approach to addiction recovery:

1. Admit you are powerless over the addiction.
2. Have faith that a higher power beyond yourself can help you.
3. Make the decision to hand over control to this higher power.
4. Always keep a personal inventory.
5. Admit to yourself, to the higher power in charge and to the others in your group any wrongs you may have done.
6. Be willing to allow your errors to be corrected by the higher power.
7. Request the higher power to remove these shortcomings.
8. Create a list of all the wrong things you may have done against others and be willing to make amends.
9. Reach out to the people you may have hurt, unless it poses a risk to their health and wellness.
10. Continue keeping an inventory and acknowledge when you hurt others.
11. Try to connect with the higher power through meditation.
12. Share these strategies with others who may need them.

In many rehabilitation centers, this twelve-step approach to addiction is often combined with evidence-based treatment that involves the use of medication. Although there are references to 'God' or a higher power in this twelve-step approach to treatment, this program is not religious. As a matter of fact, the higher power can be anything that you consider to be bigger than you.

The twelve-step approach to opioid addiction treatment and recovery provides a safe and supportive environment for recovering opioid addicts to share their experiences with others who have gone through similar struggles. In the structured therapy meetings, not only is knowledge imparted, but positive relationships are also forged. Twelve-step meetings can be found in many locations throughout the United States. Individuals who are in their early stages of recovery usually attend several meetings every week, although attendance is not always mandatory.

One of the most unique features of the twelve-step group therapy meetings is that they are typically led by individuals who have recovered from addiction instead of drug counselors. Participants are allowed and encouraged to share their experiences and perspectives with other members of their group. They are, however, strongly discouraged from speaking about the members' stories with outsiders. This ensures that the meetings maintain some level of confidentiality in order to ensure the privacy of participants is respected and upheld.

Research has shown that individuals who take part in the twelve-step approach generally tend to reduce their opioid use compared to those who do not go through this kind of therapy. Studies have also shown that early involvement in a twelve-step program can significantly increase the chances of successful long-lasting treatment.

Brief Motivational Interventions

Brief motivational interventions are short-term strategies that are put in place in order to help reduce the use of opioids by those who are dependent on them. These interventions usually entail two components namely:

- A thorough assessment of the quantity, frequency, and implications of drug use.
- Customized motivational strategies that are based on personal feedback and behavioral comparison.

Studies have shown that through a personal assessment of one's addictive actions, changes can be made to the manner in which one responds to one's urges and impulses. By gaining a deeper awareness of the risks involved in their drug use, individuals are able to develop a more balanced perspective, and effect changes that are required to stop using drugs.

Apart from the assessment of one's habitual patterns, brief motivational interventions entail the use of one or more motivational improvement strategies. This approach is predicated on the idea that the cost of addictive habits must outweigh the benefits in order for an individual to be motivated enough to change.

Medication Management

In nearly all cases of opioid addiction, treatment often involves the use of medications like methadone and buprenorphine. These drugs are usually administered to patients to neutralize the effects of opioids and reduce withdrawal symptoms that may be experienced. The aim of medication management programs is to limit the use of the drugs gradually rather than engage complete abstinence, which often produces unpleasant withdrawal symptoms.

Longer-acting opioid drugs are usually administered in this addiction treatment strategy to prevent adverse withdrawal side effects that would be induced when the agonist drug is withdrawn.

Contingency Management

Contingency management is a type of intervention that is aimed at changing one's habits through certain incentives. The guiding principle behind this treatment approach is that people are more likely to repeat certain practises if they are enforced or rewarded. There are numerous incentives that can be used in this intervention to help fight addiction. These include low-value cash incentives, gift vouchers incentives, and clinic privileges.

Studies suggest that contingency management can be very effective when it comes to promoting positive practices to people who are struggling with opioid addiction. Nevertheless, this treatment strategy has also garnered a lot of criticism from clinicians. There are those who believe that this approach is unethical since it essentially involves bribing people in order to get them to behave in ways that are ultimately beneficial for themselves. Others have even argued that the use of rewards to motivate habitual change in opioid addicts may undermine their intrinsic motivations, thus jeopardizing treatment outcomes. Finally, there are those who have raised objections purely on financial terms. They argue that this approach is too expensive and unsustainable in the long run.

Despite these objections, many addiction therapists are beginning to employ this strategy in their arsenal when it comes to treating patients who suffer from opioid addiction. When combined with other treatment approaches, contingency management can go a long way in helping an opioid-dependent change habits that fuel their addiction.

Peer Support and Lifestyle Changes

Strong peer support is very crucial during the recovery period since it provides an anchor for the individual as they go through different treatment programs and strategies. Moreover, peers can offer guidance on the strategies to apply in order to minimize the risk of relapse.

The support of friends and relatives also plays an important role in the process of addiction recovery. Remember, addiction recovery is a lifelong journey that requires a lot of patience and dedication. Unless an individual has people around them who are willing to support and care for them throughout the process, they may struggle with recovery.

Granted, living with a person who is dependent on opioids can complicate relationships by eroding trust and weakening communication. With the right support and care from close associates, people who struggle with opioid addiction can make great strides in their recovery journey. Here are some of the key ways in which the relatives and friends of recovering addicts can help them make progress in their fight against opioid addiction:

- Understand that the addiction treatment is not a quick fix, and there is a chance that the recovering patient might relapse multiple times.
- Create a healthy environment for the recovering individual by keeping the home drug-free.
- Become actively involved in the treatment and monitor the progress of the recovering patient.
- Try to learn about the recovering patient's stressors and triggers and minimize them where possible.

Dealing with a loved one's opioid addiction can undoubtedly be a very heart-wrenching experience. By providing them with the right support and being invested in their recovery, you can significantly increase their chances of achieving a complete recovery and living drug-free lives.

As we come to the end of this chapter, let us briefly recap some of the key pointers that we have discussed:

- Opioid addiction has a biological as well as mental component which must be considered when determining the right approach to treatment.
- There are several FDA-approved drugs that are crucial in the medicinal treatment of opioid dependence and addiction, including, methadone, buprenorphine and naltrexone.
- Successful treatment of opioid addiction requires a combined approach using various strategies which address the different elements that contribute to opioid dependency.
- Support from relatives, friends, and society as a whole can

significantly increase the chances of individuals making a full recovery from substance abuse and addiction.
- Cognitive-behavioral therapy along with medical interventions are necessary strategies in addiction treatment since they help the recovering patient recognize and change the negative behaviors which contribute to their disease.

8

TMC AND OTHER NATURAL TREATMENTS

Most medical and behavioral interventions that are used for opioid addiction treatments are highly effective at helping individuals overcome the habit. These interventions do come with their fair share of side effects, most of which can be very difficult to contend with. The use of opioid antagonists like methadone, naloxone, and buprenorphine, for instance, produces withdrawal effects which are very unpleasant. In light of this, it is prudent to consider alternative pain-management treatments that are available in case you are struggling with opioid dependence and addiction.

In this closing chapter, we will investigate a number of alternative treatments for addiction, including traditional Chinese medicine, acupuncture and acupressure, herbs, essential oils, and flower essence. By the end of this topic, you will have all that you require in order to make the right choice when it comes to the most suitable supplemental treatments to boost your recovery.

Before we begin, let me reiterate that the strategies and products outlined here should be used in conjunction with approved treatments for opioid addiction, as they are designed to help ease the transition from dependency to recovery by enhancing the physical and emotional state of the individual.

Traditional Chinese Medicine (TCM)

For thousands of years, traditional Chinese medicine has been used to treat a wide array of conditions, including mental illnesses and drug addiction. One of the concepts used to assess the problem of addiction is known as the 'empty flare,' which presupposes that the flaring up of behavioral and emotional symptoms of addiction is a result of the loss of a calm center. The treatment is designed to restore balance and nourish the Yin aspect in order to facilitate recovery.

TCM approaches to addiction treatment typically encapsulate the entire process of recovery from the time the problem is diagnosed to the time an individual has fully recovered from their drug dependence. This natural treatment strategy works to support the patient through the withdrawal process by helping to minimize the effects and reduce cravings. TCM aims to treat opioid addiction without the use of the antagonist drugs that are commonly employed in Western approaches to treatment.

Acupuncture and Acupressure

Acupuncture is one of the most common all-natural therapies that is employed in the treatment of opioid addiction as well as other health problems like back pain, fibromyalgia, and headaches. This technique was developed thousands of years ago and has since been adopted in many regions around the world. What is acupuncture and how is it used to treat addiction?

Acupuncture is a non-drug therapy that involves the stimulation of various body points using needles to relieve or eliminate physical and mental pain. Since the early 1970s, acupuncture has been an integral part of treatments designed to alleviate stress, anxiety, depression and drug addiction. It involves sticking needles into the bodies of patients to help ease the withdrawal symptoms that are associated with substance addiction. Studies have shown that patients who undergo this type of therapy in addition to other comprehensive treatments like psychological counseling, peer-group support involvement, and education experience a number of benefits, including reduced drug cravings, better quality of sleep, and relief from anxiety.

How effective is acupuncture when it comes to opioid addiction treatment? Numerous studies have been conducted to determine the success rate of acupuncture as a treatment for opioid dependence and addiction. In one particular study, auricular acupuncture was used to treat 82 patients struggling with cocaine addiction. The subjects were administered daily acupuncture treatment sessions for a period of two months. The findings showed that patients who received these treatments along with medical therapies using drugs like methadone were more likely to abstain from cocaine use compared to patients who were only treated with methadone.

Similar studies have been conducted on patients struggling with other forms of addiction, including alcohol and tobacco. The positive findings of these studies seem to suggest that acupuncture can be used in the treatment of opioid addiction. This treatment is most effective when combined with other therapies such as behavioral counseling and medical interventions.

In order to gauge the appropriateness of acupuncture for a patient's needs, it is important for the nature and structure of this treatment to be understood. This allows the patient to know what to expect with this type of therapy and prepare both physically and mentally for the treatment. The initial step in acupuncture treatment typically entails examining a person's health history, their timeline of addiction, and any underlying physical and mental illnesses. The therapist may also ask about any physical pain or stress that the patient may be experiencing.

Once the medical history of the patient has been established, the doctor will conduct a medical examination to establish the severity of their addiction before providing a referral to an acupuncture therapist. After the therapist has performed a thorough assessment of your physical and psychological health, they will prescribe a variety of acupuncture treatments to get rid of physical pain and make you more relaxed. Treatment typically entails inserting needles through various pressure points on the body. This procedure should be done slowly and carefully to minimize the potential for pain. Usually, the needles are left on the skin for between five to thirty minutes.

In some cases, the needles may need to be heated or twirled in order to maximize their effectiveness. Once the recommended therapy time has elapsed, the needles are carefully removed from the skin and ointment is applied to soothe the pain. The treatment may be administered several times a week depending on the needs of the patient.

Although acupuncture has been proven to be very beneficial in reversing the effects of drug use, it is not recommended as a single therapy for opioid addiction. This is mainly because recovering patients may still need to go through a medical detoxification process to boost their chances of full recovery.

Acupressure is a natural treatment technique which is very similar to acupuncture. Unlike acupuncture which involves the application of needles into specific parts of the body, acupressure generally involves the use of fingertips to manually apply pressure on key points. The application of acupressure is believed to help alleviate pain by stimulating the production of feel-good hormones known as endorphins. Consequently, acupressure can be used to manage chronic pain arising due to medical conditions such as menstrual cramps, muscle tension, nausea induced by chemotherapy, and many other illnesses.

The greatest benefits of acupuncture and acupressure in opioid addiction treatment lies in their ability to relieve pain and promote relaxation. These techniques can help alleviate the mental and emotional distress associated with opioid addiction. Hence, by combining them

HERBS

Herbal therapies are often employed in the treatment of substance addiction and dependence. These treatments are not meant to be stand-alone addiction recovery therapies; they are used in conjunction with other treatment strategies to improve the success rate of addiction treatment. Some of the most popular plant-based medicines include:

Hawthorne Berries

Hawthorne berries have been shown to be highly beneficial for hearts that have been weakened by prolonged substance abuse and eating disorders such as bulimia and anorexia. These berries are generally mild in their composition, and consequently pose no threat to individuals whose cardiovascular health has been undermined by prolonged opioid abuse.

It usually takes several weeks of daily use before the effects of this powerful natural herbal medicine become apparent. In case you prefer to avoid the alcohol-content in this herbal plant, you can simply put your dosage of the herb in boiling water for a few minutes. This will cause the alcohol composition to evaporate so that you are left with pure medicine.

Dandelion

Prolonged usage of opioid substances can cause significant damage to the spleen, which is responsible for protecting the body against infections and keeping body fluids in balance. Although this herb is safe to use, you should take extra caution, especially if you are suffering from gallstones.

Milk Thistle

Milk thistle is a strong herbal medicine that can help soothe the liver in case it has been damaged by continual opioid use. This herbal plant improves the ability of the liver to eliminate drugs and other harmful chemicals, thereby making it a highly beneficial medicine to include in any comprehensive addiction recovery plan. It should be noted that this herbal extract may induce mild diarrhea since it stimulates the production of bile but should not be a serious cause for concern. In case you experience this unpleasant side effect, you should simply take a break from the medicine until your bowel movements normalize, and then increase the dose gradually over time.

Burdock Root

Burdock root is a natural herb that acts as an anti-inflammatory agent, an antioxidant, and a blood purifier. It also functions as a diuretic by stimulating the body's release of excess water and flushing chemical compounds from the body through the kidneys. In addition to this, burdock root is also a nutritive herb that helps replenish the body with nutrients that may have been flushed out by dysfunctional kidneys.

Regular intake of burdock root allows your body to heal during the addiction recovery process, and should be a part of your daily herbal protocol. For best results, you may want to combine it with camomile, lemon balm, and basil.

MEDITATION THERAPY

Meditation is a very powerful and simple technique that has been proven to be highly effective in treating a wide array of mental and emotional health issues including depression, anxiety, and stress. In recent years, the practice of meditation has also been co-opted as a strategy for treating drug and substance addiction. Earlier on, we discussed some of the psychological implications of opioid abuse on mental health and saw the complex relationship of dual diagnosis disorders which encompass both drug addiction and mental illness. It is only logical, then, that treatments for addiction also envisage the mental wellbeing of people who are trying to recover from opioid addiction.

The aim of meditation therapy is to enable the individual to foster a sense of balance between their physical and mental states. Meditation techniques such as breathing exercises and mantra chants can help increase an individual's awareness and make them become more connected. Some of the characteristics which are commonly associated with all meditative practices include the lotus pose and controlled breathing exercises. There are various methods of meditation therapy that are designed to benefit individuals in specific ways. These include:

Mindfulness Meditation

This is the ability of an individual to be fully aware of what is going on within them as well as in their external environment without being overly reactive or overwhelmed. Individuals who are able to exercise mindfulness meditation are more capable of coping with the withdrawal symptoms of opioids without relapsing back to dependence and addiction. Moreover, it can help reduce anxiety and depression, providing recovering opioid users with the mental strength and fortitude that they require in order to completely give up the habit of substance abuse.

Zen Meditation

This is a form of meditation that is rooted in ancient Buddhist psychology and philosophy. The aim of this meditation method is to regulate an individual's attention through a practice known as "thinking about not thinking." Zen meditation usually requires practitioners to sit in a lotus position (with their legs crossed) and focus their attention inwards. Sometimes, it may also include controlled breathing exercises in which the practitioner keeps count of their inhales and exhales.

The practice of Zen meditation is quite similar to mindfulness meditation since it is aimed at cultivating a presence of mind. Unlike mindfulness, whose objective it is to focus one's attention on a particular object, Zen meditation is meant to foster general awareness. Individuals who practice this form of meditation are able to expand the scope of their attention and increase their awareness of their thoughts, emotions, and perceptions

Studies have shown that Zen meditation offers numerous cognitive, emotional and physical benefits to its practitioners. Apart from alleviating symptoms of stress and anxiety, it can also help recovering opioid addicts to become more connected and aware of their personal predispositions. This can influence them to let go of destructive thought patterns and actions that trigger their addictive tendencies and allow them to form positive thought and behavioral patterns that will catalyze their recovery.

Guided Meditation

Guided meditation is a form of relaxed meditative practice that is led by another person known as a teacher. The guide in this type of meditation can be a spiritual guru, yoga instructor or even a recorded CD. The role of the guide is to narrate the dynamics of the mind during meditation and instruct the individual on how to perform the meditation techniques.

If you are looking to start practicing this form of meditation therapy, you may need to enroll for a meditation class. If you live in a city or town where finding an instructor is difficult, there are various mobile apps that you can use to perform guided meditation by yourself in the comfort of your home.

There are plenty of benefits that guided meditation offers to those who practice. These include increased awareness, reduced negative thinking, and increased ability to cope with stressful situations and increased tolerance for pain and discomfort - this is particularly important for people who are trying to quit prescription opioids and adopt healthier ways of dealing with chronic pain. Guided meditation can also help those who are struggling with opioid addiction to become more mentally resilient in order to follow through with treatment despite the negative withdrawal effects that they may experience during abstinence.

Transcendental Meditation

This is a method of meditation that is aimed at cultivating and maintaining a state of relaxed awareness. During the practice of transcendental meditation, the practitioner is required to sit in a comfortable position with their eyes closed and recite a mantra that allows them to focus their concentration.

Through this process, the ordinary awareness of the individual is transcended, and they are able to achieve a state of pure consciousness or 'being.' At this point, the practitioner reaches a state of perfect stillness, stability, and order, unaffected by whatever bodily sensations or emotions they may be experiencing.

Transcendental meditation has been shown to offer impressive health benefits to those who pursue it. This form of meditation therapy can help reduce chronic pain, relieve anxiety and depression, improve immunity, and promote overall well being. Individuals who struggle with opioid addiction can greatly benefit from incorporating this therapy in whatever treatments they are already undergoing.

ESSENTIAL OILS

Essential oils have been shown to offer numerous benefits when it comes to addiction recovery. Although these products do not function as cures for addiction, they can provide a much-needed boost to one's mental health and promote overall wellness in the long run. Essential oils are usually employed in a treatment known as aromatherapy. Here are some of the ways in which the use of essential oils can improve the process of recovery from addiction:

- They help reduce withdrawal symptoms once an individual cuts on opioid use.
- They minimize anxiety and stress.
- They can improve one's mood.
- They induce relaxation and can help improve the quality of sleep.
- They help in alleviating chronic pain.
- They can significantly boost one's immune system.
- They can provide mental clarity and peace.

There are various essential oils that can be used in addiction recovery treatments, including:

Ginger Oil

This essential oil is usually extracted from the rhizomes of the ginger plant through a distillation process. It has a strong scent, spicy and warm. Ginger oil is commonly used in aromatherapy, and has been shown to have several benefits to its users, including alleviating headaches and providing relief from arthritis pain. It can also help soothe nausea, which is one of the main symptoms associated with opioid use and abuse.

Grapefruit Oil

Grapefruit oil is an orange-tinted essential oil, which is extracted from the peels of the grapefruit through a process known as cold-pressing. This citrus-scented oil is often used in aromatherapy thanks to the myriads of benefits that it offers. Grapefruit oil produces a calming effect on the body and mind, relieves anxiety and stress and lowers blood pressure. In addition to these health benefits, studies have shown that this essential oil also has mood stabilizing properties that can help reduce intense cravings. It is not surprising that many health and wellness experts often recommend Grapefruit oil to people who are trying to kick the habit of opioid use.

Bergamot Oil

Bergamot is an essential oil that is derived from the rinds of citrus fruits that grow on the Bergamot orange plant. This compound is highly prized for its natural sweet scent, and lends itself to a wide variety of applications. Bergamot oil is also known to produce a number of benefits including stress reduction, anti-inflammation, and pain relief.

The oil can be applied in various ways such as room diffusion and skin application. When used as an ointment, bergamot oil should be diluted with a carrier oil to prevent skin irritation.

TREATING OPIOID DEPENDENCE BY CORRECTING ELEMENTAL BALANCES

In Chinese Medicine, there are five natural elements in nature that correspond to the energies that move through the life force of an individual. These fundamental elements are wood, fire, metal earth, and water. It is thought that for an individual to be healthy, these elemental forces must be in balance. Each of the elements corresponds to or is associated with a particular energy point or body part. For instance, wood symbolizes the liver and gallbladder, fire represents the heart, earth is associated with the spleen, metal denotes the lungs, and water represents the kidneys.

When one or more of these elements are not balanced in the body, an individual may become prone to sickness. As a result, treatment is often aimed at restoring the balance of these crucial life forces. The diagnostic approach in this Traditional form of medicine is usually very thorough. In addition to conducting blood sugar and cholesterol tests, the medical practitioner may also ask the patient questions to determine their sensory experience. Depending on the symptoms presented, the doctor will then probe deeper to determine the elemental imbalance that is causing the symptoms

Treatment plans in this form of medicine are usually highly customized, and may include detoxification, clinical nutrition, and the use of Chinese medicinal herbs.

There are plenty of natural therapies that can be applied concurrently with clinical interventions when treating opioid addiction. Here are the main takeaways from this chapter on how these non-drug treatments should be applied:

- Traditional Chinese Medicine (TCM) therapies can be used to boost one's physical and mental resolve to quit opioid use, thereby increasing their chances of recovery.
- Acupuncture is very effective at treating chronic pain and can be applied as an alternative pain-relief treatment to prescription opioids.
- Various herbs such as Hawthorne berries and dandelions help reverse the effect of prolonged opioid use and facilitate faster recovery of organs that have been affected by addiction.
- Essential oils can help alleviate the serious withdrawal effects that arise from opioid addiction, thus improving the chances of full recovery.
- All-natural treatments must be used in conjunction with medication therapies and psychological counseling in order to provide holistic treatment for opioid addiction.

AFTERWORD

Drug and substance abuse is without a doubt one of the biggest challenges that our society has been facing in recent history. The increased use of prescription opioids and similar illegal drugs has unwittingly given rise to a new drug crisis which we are far from solving. Policymakers have often asserted that drug addiction is a criminal matter that requires legal recourse to defeat it. Nevertheless, the failure of public policy to rein in opioid addiction is proof that we need to rethink our strategy if we are to defeat this enemy.

My aim for writing this book was two-fold. First, I wanted to give voice to a more objective perspective on addiction, based not only on anecdotal evidence but also on scientific case studies. The prevailing attitudes towards substance abuse and addiction have always been very reductionist and contemptuous. Individuals who struggle with drug addiction are always seen as weak-minded, and their suffering is usually chalked up to poor life choices. An even more cynical attitude presumes that those who are addicted or dependent on these substances actually take them simply because they enjoy doing so. This, however, is not only a false deduction but can actually be a very destructive mindset. We have seen how false perceptions such as these often fuel stigma against persons who are struggling with addiction and make it difficult for them to access the treatment they require in order to kick the habit.

The fact of the matter is that addiction is not a result of poor choices or weak will. On the contrary, it is a chronic illness that requires continual comprehensive treatment and care to overcome. We have seen how complex and multi-layered this illness is, in the sense that it not only affects one's physical health but can also have significant implications for a person's psychological state. To achieve full recovery, treatment should focus not only on restoring the physical health of the patient but also on improving their mental health so that they are able to abstain from drug use altogether.

My other objective for writing this book, which is perhaps more important, is to provide effective treatment strategies that can be employed in the fight against addiction. Due to a lack of information about the dynamics of this crisis, many people often wrongly assume that individuals who are dependent on drugs can quit using them if they simply decide to do so. This perception is very ill-informed, since it fails to account for actions that contribute to perpetual opioid dependence and addiction. We have seen how prolonged opioid use leads to changes in brain chemistry, which can alter not only one's mood but their ability to control and regulate their behavior. Obviously, there is an element of individual choice during the initial stage of opioid use. Once individuals develop tolerance and dependence, however, it can be very difficult for them to give up the use of opioids due to the adverse symptoms that are occasioned by withdrawal.

As such, the right treatment strategy should focus on helping the person gradually cut down on their opioid use until they reach a point of complete abstinence. Opioid antagonists like buprenorphine, methadone, and naloxone have been approved by the FDA for use in addiction treatment programs. These highly effective drugs are known to work by attaching to the brain's receptors in the same way that opioids do, thereby reversing the effects of agonists like morphine, codeine and heroin. Despite the effectiveness of these drugs, they may also produce unpleasant side effects, which can complicate treatment and make recovery much more difficult.

To improve the chances for successful recovery, these medical therapies should be combined with other strategies. One of the most important therapies that can be used together with medical interventions is psychological counseling. Since substance addiction often manifests together with mental illness in the form of a dual diagnosis, failure to employ holistic treatment for both conditions may lead to a cycle of addiction and poor mental health.

To slay the beast of dual diagnosis disorders, patients require behavioral therapy that trains them on how to identify the negative automatic thoughts that contribute to addictive practices. Behavioral therapy also enables recovering patients to learn positive coping mechanisms that can help them follow through with their treatment despite the challenging withdrawal symptoms that they may experience. In addition to the approved treatment strategies for addiction, there are a number of natural therapies that can be applied to alleviate the symptoms of addiction. These include Traditional Chinese Medicine and therapies such as acupuncture and acupressure, the use of herbs and essential oils as well as mental health therapies like meditation and yoga. While these natural methods do not single-handedly cure the illness, combined they can provide significant relief from the negative effects of opioid use and greatly boost the chances of full recovery.

We have also looked at the important role that support from peers and relatives play in opioid addiction recovery. Many individuals who struggle with opioid addictions often have very complicated relationships with their family members, friends, spouses, and community. They are often ostracized by the people closest to them, and this may take a serious toll on the victim's psychological state, and even trigger anxiety and depression.

On the other hand, when patients are provided with care, support and love, they are more likely to go through treatment successfully, and fully recover from their drug problem. To help our loved ones and friends to quit the habit of opioid use, it is vital that we invest our efforts towards their recovery, be patient with them, care for them, and support them throughout the process. Granted, living with a person who is recovering from opioid use can be psychologically and emotionally straining for the affected person. Persevering with them throughout the recovery process even when they relapse can lead to a better understanding of each other can in turn foster growth in relationships.

In conclusion, I would like to reiterate that although opioid addiction is a serious disease that can have negative effects on every aspect of one's life, it is not automatically a death sentence. Tens of thousands of people have been able to fully recover from opioid addiction, and have gone on to live productive lives. If you are struggling with substance addiction, you need not lose hope of recovery. With the right treatment, support and guidance, you too can kick the habit of opioid addiction and begin living a healthy and productive life once more.

In this book, I have painstakingly outlined answers to ending substance abuse and how to give up an opioid addiction. I have no doubt in my mind that you will find the wisdom contained herein very useful as you struggle to overcome the problem of addiction. In case you have loved ones who are trying to kick their opioid use, don't hesitate to share the knowledge you have received in this guide with them. You never know: it just might be the turning point that causes them to rethink their lives and make positive changes.

Finally, I would like to thank everyone who has been an invaluable help in the arduous yet very satisfying journey of writing this book. I do not underestimate the important insights that I have received from the respondents, experts, and patients that I have worked within the course of researching this subject. I would also like to thank you for choosing this book. I hope it has been an enjoyable and highly informative read. Kindly give us a review and share what you think about this book and what you have learned from it.

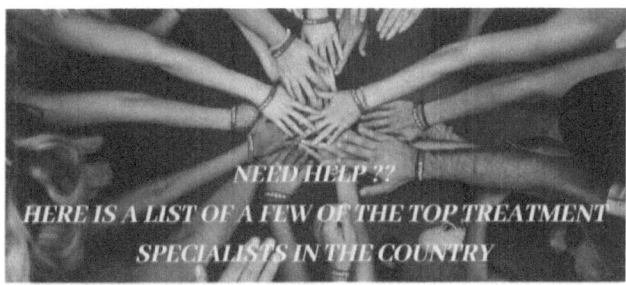

THE LIST INCLUDES:

- *Nationally renowned treatment providers*
- *One-click linked portal access*
- *Locations and contact information*
- *Things to remember when seeking or providing help*

It's one thing to need help, and another to know where to go......

To receive your Renowned Treatment List, visit the link:

Renowned Treatment List

REFERENCES

A. (2017, December 11). Different Types and Causes of Substance Abuse - San Diego | API. Retrieved from https://apibhs.com/2017/12/11/types-causes-of-substance-abuse

Arjan, A. (2018, June 19). How Does Drug Addiction Affect Relationships? Retrieved from https://medmark.com/how-does-drug-addiction-affect-relationships/

Assistant Secretary of Public Affairs (ASPA). (2018, April 19). Treatment for Opioid Use Disorder and Addiction. Retrieved from https://www.hhs.gov/opioids/treatment/index.html

Body In Mind Archives. (n.d.). Retrieved April 26, 2020, from https://relief.news/category/body-in-mind/

Bueno-Gómez, N. (2017, September 29). Conceptualizing suffering and pain. Retrieved from https://peh-med.biomedcentral.com/articles/10.1186/s13010-017-0049-5

Butanis, B. (2018, April 30). What Are Opioids? Retrieved from https://www.hopkinsmedicine.org/opioids/what-are-opioids.html

Division, D. C. (2018, November 21). Prevention Programs & Tools. Retrieved from https://www.hhs.gov/opioids/prevention/prevention-programs-tools/index.html

Drug addiction (substance use disorder) - Symptoms and causes. (2017, October 26). Retrieved from https://www.mayoclinic.org/diseases-conditions/drug-addiction/symptoms-causes/syc-20365112

Drug, Alcohol Addiction: What are the Factors That Play a Role? (2020, March 5). Retrieved from https://emeraldcoastjourneypure.com/drug-alcohol-addiction-factors/

Felman, A. (2018, November 2). What are the treatments for addiction? Retrieved from https://www.medicalnewstoday.com/articles/323468#counseling-and-behavioral

Franchini, A. (2020, January 22). Opiate vs. Opioid – Do You Know the Difference? Retrieved from https://recoverycentersofamerica.com/blogs/opiate-vs-opioid-do-you-know-the-difference/

Genetics Home Reference. (n.d.). Opioid addiction. Retrieved April 26, 2020, from https://ghr.nlm.nih.gov/condition/opioid-addiction

Harvard Health Publishing. (2011, July 1). How addiction hijacks the brain. Retrieved from https://www.health.harvard.edu/newsletter_article/how-addiction-hijacks-the-brain

History of Pain: A Brief Overview of the 19th and 20th Centuries. (n.d.). Retrieved April 26, 2020, from https://www.practicalpainmanagement.com/treatments/history-pain-brief-overview-19th-20th-centuries

History of the Opioid Epidemic. (2018, August 16). Retrieved from https://dualdiagnosis.org/infographics/history-of-the-opioid-epidemic/

How opioid addiction occurs. (2018, February 16). Retrieved from https://www.mayoclinic.org/diseases-conditions/prescription-drug-abuse/in-depth/how-opioid-addiction-occurs/art-20360372

Juergens, J. (2019, December 6). Opiate Addiction, Abuse and Treatment. Retrieved from https://www.addictioncenter.com/opiates/

Lallanilla, M. (2006, January 6). A Brief History of Pain. Retrieved from https://abcnews.go.com/Health/PainManagement/story?id=731553&page=1

National Institute on Drug Abuse. (n.d.). A Letter to Parents. Retrieved April 26, 2020, from https://www.drugabuse.gov/publications/opioids-facts-parents-need-to-know/letter-to-parents

Northwestern Medicine. (2018, March 23). What You Need to Know About Opioids. Retrieved from https://www.nm.org/healthbeat/healthy-tips/what-you-need-to-know-about-opioids

Pain (Stanford Encyclopedia of Philosophy). (2019, March 4). Retrieved from https://plato.stanford.edu/entries/pain/

pubmeddev. (n.d.). Clonidine and naltrexone. A safe, effective, and rapid treatment of abrupt withdrawal from methadone therapy. - PubMed - NCBI. Retrieved April 26, 2020, from https://www.ncbi.nlm.nih.gov/pubmed/7138234

Stigma of Addiction | Reducing the Stigma of Substance Abuse. (2019, February 21). Retrieved from https://drugabuse.com/addiction/stigma/

TEDx Talks. (2018, November 26). The Stigma of Addiction | Tony Hoffman | TEDxFresnoState. Retrieved from https://www.youtube.com/watch?v=FuooVrSpffk

TEDx Talks. (2019, June 24). Shaming the Sick: Substance Use and Stigma | Dr Carolyn Greer | TEDxFortWayne. Retrieved from https://www.youtube.com/watch?v=eZ0CafocLsY

The Cause & Effect of Substance Abuse & Mental Health Issues. (2020, March 23). Retrieved from https://sunrisehouse.com/cause-effect/

The Neurobiology of Opioid Dependence: Implications for Treatment. (2002, July 1). Retrieved from https://www.ncbi.nlm.nih.gov/pmc/articles/PMC2851054/

The role of lifestyle in perpetuating substance use disorder: the Lifestyle Balance Model. (2020, April 26). Retrieved from https://www.ncbi.nlm.nih.gov/pmc/articles/PMC4326198/

What Are Opioids? - When Seconds Count. (n.d.). Retrieved April 26, 2020, from https://www.asahq.org/whensecondscount/pain-management/opioid-treatment/what-are-opioids/

What are the biggest misconceptions around addiction? (n.d.). Retrieved April 26, 2020, from https://www.drugrehab.com/addiction/stigma/

What causes addiction? (2018, November 2). Retrieved from https://www.medicalnewstoday.com/articles/323483#takeaway

What Causes Addiction? The Science of Drug & Alcohol Addictions. (2019, June 12). Retrieved from https://drugabuse.com/causes-of-addiction/

Wikipedia contributors. (2019, November 25). The body in traditional Chinese medicine. Retrieved from https://en.wikipedia.org/wiki/The_body_in_traditional_Chinese_medicine

Wikipedia contributors. (2020, April 14). Pain theories. Retrieved from https://en.wikipedia.org/wiki/Pain_theories

www.ingramcontent.com/pod-product-compliance
Lightning Source LLC
Chambersburg PA
CBHW022007120526
44592CB00034B/531